101 WESTERN Short Stories For Seniors

Short Stories for Seniors 3

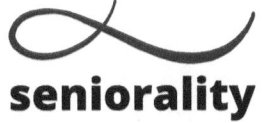

1. Desert Vendetta

In the shadow of the setting sun, dust kicked up like smoke from the hooves of his horse as the gunslinger rode into the desolate town of Deadwood. His name was Ethan Cole, a man forged by tragedy and fueled by vengeance. The memory of that fateful night haunted him, the screams of his wife and son echoing in his mind like a relentless storm.

It had been six months since the outlaw gang, led by the notorious Dalton brothers, had mercilessly gunned down his family in cold blood. Now, Ethan's heart burned with a singular purpose: to track down those responsible and make them pay.

As he dismounted in front of the dusty saloon, Ethan's steely gaze swept across the faces of the townsfolk, their eyes avoiding his own. They knew who he was and what he sought, but none dared to stand in his way.

Inside the dimly lit saloon, the air was thick with the smell of whiskey and cigar smoke. The sound of a poker game echoed from the back room, mingling with the raucous laughter of the patrons. Ethan's hand instinctively went to the handle of his Colt revolver as he made his way through the crowd.

The Dalton brothers were holed up in the back room, surrounded by their lackeys and counting their ill-gotten gains. But when Ethan burst through the door, his presence silenced the room like a sudden clap of thunder.

Without a word, Ethan drew his gun and leveled it at the eldest Dalton brother. "You took everything from me," he growled, his voice low and dangerous. "Now it's time to pay the price."

The room erupted into chaos as gunfire filled the air, but Ethan remained steady, his aim unwavering. In the end, justice would be served, one bullet at a time.

2. The Wild Heart of Calamity Jane

Her name was Martha Canary, but to the world, she was known as Calamity Jane.

With fiery red hair and a spirit as wild as the land itself, Calamity Jane was a force to be reckoned with—a sharpshooter, a horsewoman, and a legend in her own right. From the saloons of Deadwood to the dusty trails of the Dakota Territory, she roamed the land with a sense of freedom and adventure that captivated all who crossed her path.

But behind the fearless exterior lay a woman haunted by her own demons, a woman whose heart longed for something more than the transient thrills of the frontier. Beneath the bravado and swagger, there lurked a vulnerability that few ever glimpsed—a vulnerability born of a turbulent past and a longing for belonging.

It was amidst the chaos of the Wild West that Calamity Jane's legend truly began to take shape. With her trusty rifle at her side and a band of misfits by her side, she embarked on a series of daring escapades that would become the stuff of legend—a stagecoach robbery here, a showdown with outlaws there, each adventure more thrilling than the last.

But amidst the chaos and excitement, there was one constant in Calamity Jane's life—a man named Wild Bill Hickok. Theirs was a bond forged in the crucible of the frontier, a bond that transcended mere friendship and bloomed into something deeper—a love that burned as fiercely as the prairie sun.

Yet theirs was a love doomed from the start, a love torn apart by fate and circumstance. And as Calamity Jane rode off into the sunset, her heart heavy with sorrow, she knew that she would always carry a piece of Wild Bill with her—a piece of the man who had captured her heart and forever changed the course of her life.

For Calamity Jane was more than just a legend—she was a woman of courage and conviction, a woman whose wild spirit would live on in history for generations to come.

3. Outlaw's Gambit

In the unforgiving desert, under the scorching sun, a band of outlaws gathered in the dimly lit backroom of the Last Chance Saloon. They were a motley crew of desperados, each with their own dark past and a thirst for adventure.

Their leader, a hardened gunslinger known only as Gravedigger, leaned back in his chair, his steely gaze fixed on the map spread out before them. The plan was simple yet daring: to rob the First National Bank of Red Rock, the largest and most heavily guarded bank in the territory.

As the outlaws debated the finer details of their scheme, tensions ran high. The risks were great, and the stakes even greater. But for Gravedigger and his men, the lure of the ultimate heist was too tantalizing to resist.

Under the cover of darkness, they rode out into the night, their horses kicking up clouds of dust as they galloped across the desert plains. With nerves of steel and guns at the ready, they approached the imposing stone walls of the bank.

As they burst through the doors, guns blazing, chaos erupted in the streets of Red Rock. The sound of gunfire echoed through the night as the outlaws made their way to the vault, overcoming every obstacle in their path.

But just as victory seemed within their grasp, disaster struck. The sheriff and his posse arrived, guns drawn and ready for battle. In a desperate bid to escape, Gravedigger and his men fought tooth and nail, their bullets flying fast and furious.

In the end, only Gravedigger remained standing, the sole survivor of the ill-fated heist. As he rode off into the sunset, his pockets weighed down with gold, he knew that the price of his freedom would be steep. But for a true outlaw, the thrill of the chase was worth any cost.

4. The Dust Settles

In the arid expanse of the Southwest, beneath the relentless glare of the sun, Caleb Houston rode alone. His only companions were the wind and the rhythmic hoofbeats of his steed. A veteran bounty hunter, Caleb had faced down many a desperado, but none had haunted him like the man he now hunted: Jeb "Ironhand" McCallister.

Jeb was a shadow, rumored to have more kills to his name than the stars in the desert sky. His reign of terror had left a trail of blood across the territory, and now it was Caleb's duty to bring him to justice.

As Caleb rode, the memories of Jeb's crimes weighed heavy on his mind. He recalled the faces of the innocent victims, their families torn apart by senseless violence. Determination burned in his chest like a wildfire as he vowed to see justice served.

After days of relentless pursuit, Caleb finally caught up to his quarry in a dusty canyon. The two men faced each other, their eyes locking in silent recognition. Jeb sneered, his hand twitching toward the gun at his hip, but Caleb was quicker.

In a heartbeat, the air was filled with the deafening roar of gunfire. Bullets whistled through the air, kicking up clouds of dust as Caleb and Jeb exchanged lead. The shootout seemed to stretch on for an eternity, but in the end, there could only be one victor. When the dust settled, Caleb emerged victorious, his chest heaving with exertion. With Jeb's lifeless body at his feet, Caleb felt a sense of closure wash over him. The chapter of Jeb McCallister was finally closed, and justice had been served in the unforgiving landscape of the Wild West.

5. Trail of Endurance

Jed and his fellow cowhands drove their herd along the dusty trail that led across the rugged plains. It was supposed to be a routine cattle drive, but nothing was ever routine in the unforgiving wilderness.

One night, a ferocious storm struck, driving the cattle into a panicked frenzy. Lightning split the sky, and thunder boomed like a cannonade. In the chaos, a stampede ensued, tearing through the camp and scattering the men.

Jed fought to regain control, but the herd was unstoppable. In the mayhem, his horse bolted, leaving him stranded and alone. With gritted teeth, he vowed to survive, no matter the cost.

Days turned into weeks as Jed navigated the harsh terrain, his supplies dwindling with each passing mile. He faced relentless obstacles: treacherous ravines, thirst that burned like fire, and predators lurking in the shadows.

But Jed was no stranger to hardship. Born and raised in the wild, he had learned to adapt, to endure. With grim determination, he pressed on, driven by the desire to see another sunrise.

Finally, on the brink of collapse, Jed stumbled upon a small homestead nestled in a secluded valley. The weary rancher who lived there took him in, offering food, shelter, and a chance to rest his weary bones.

As Jed sat by the fire, nursing a steaming cup of coffee, he reflected on his harrowing journey. He had faced death and lived to tell the tale, proving that in the wild west, survival was not just a matter of luck—it was a test of strength, resilience, and sheer willpower.

6. Shadow on Blueridge

The town of Blueridge lay quiet, its dusty streets empty save for the occasional tumbleweed rolling by. The locals were used to the solitude, but their routine was disrupted when a stranger rode into town on a horse as black as midnight.

He wore a long duster coat that billowed in the hot wind, and his hat shaded his eyes, leaving his face hidden in shadow. The townsfolk watched with wary curiosity as he hitched his horse outside the saloon and stepped inside.

The stranger's arrival brought whispers of speculation. Some said he was running from the law, while others claimed he was searching for someone. But no one knew for sure, and none dared to ask.

As the evening wore on, the stranger kept to himself, nursing a drink at the bar while he listened to the conversations around him. His silence only fueled the rumors, and tension hung thick in the air.

But it wasn't until the next morning that the truth was revealed. The stranger's dark secret came to light when a wanted poster appeared on the sheriff's office wall, bearing his likeness and a hefty bounty.

The townsfolk were shocked, but they knew better than to challenge him. With a grim determination, the stranger mounted his horse and rode out of town, leaving behind a trail of unanswered questions and whispered rumors. And as the dust settled in his wake, the people of Blueridge were left to wonder what other secrets lay hidden in the vast expanse of the western frontier.

7. The Last Stand of John Callahan

The sun hung high over the vast plains of the West as John Callahan squinted at the distant figures riding towards his homestead. He knew them well—the hired guns of the ruthless cattle baron, Silas McLeod.

With a weary sigh, John reached for his rifle, its worn stock a testament to the battles it had seen. He was a man of the land, born and bred on these acres, and he wouldn't let some greedy baron trample over his legacy.

As the riders drew nearer, their intentions clear, John's resolve hardened. He stood tall, his weathered face a mask of determination. Behind him, the ranch hands prepared for the impending showdown, their nerves taut but their loyalty unwavering.

"McLeod!" John's voice carried across the plain, cutting through the tense silence. "This land ain't for sale, and I'll be damned if I let you take it by force."

McLeod's men laughed, their jeers echoing across the open expanse. But John remained steadfast, his grip tightening on the rifle as he stared down the barrel at his adversaries.

The standoff lasted mere moments, but to John, it felt like an eternity. Then, with a thunderous crack, the first shot rang out, signaling the start of the skirmish.

Bullets flew, and men fell, but John fought with the ferocity of a lion defending its pride. His ranch was more than just land—it was his home, his heritage, and he would protect it at any cost.

When the dust settled, John stood victorious, bloodied but unbowed. The cattle barons had been vanquished, their greed no match for his unwavering resolve. And as the sun dipped below the horizon, casting long shadows across the land, John knew that his ranch would endure, a testament to the spirit of the West.

8. The Rush for Riches

Riches buried beneath the earth stirred the souls of men, igniting a feverish frenzy known as the Gold Rush. The once quiet town of Prospectors' Hollow was thrust into chaos as prospectors from far and wide descended upon its dusty streets, their eyes gleaming with the promise of untold wealth.

Among them were lifelong friends, Ben and Tom, who had shared dreams of striking it rich since they were boys. But as the rush for gold reached a fever pitch, their bond was tested like never before.

Driven by the lure of fortune, Ben threw caution to the wind, staking claim after claim in a reckless bid for wealth and glory. Meanwhile, Tom remained steadfast, urging his friend to tread carefully and remember the values they had always held dear.

As weeks turned into months, tensions mounted and fortunes shifted. Ben's reckless pursuits yielded little more than disappointment and debt, while Tom's patience and perseverance began to pay off.

But as the gold rush reached its zenith, tragedy struck. A dispute over a lucrative claim erupted into violence, pitting friend against friend in a bitter struggle for control.

In the end, Ben's greed proved his undoing, driving a wedge between him and Tom that could never be mended. As the dust settled and the town returned to its quiet existence, Tom stood alone among the ruins of their friendship, his heart heavy with regret for what could have been.

For in the end, the true treasure of the Gold Rush was not the wealth unearthed from the earth, but the bonds of friendship and loyalty that endured, even in the face of greed and betrayal.

9. Defenders of the Land

High atop the rugged cliffs, the Lakota tribe made their stand against the encroaching settlers. For generations, they had lived in harmony with the land, honoring the spirits of the earth and sky. But now, as the iron horse thundered across the plains and the smoke of progress choked the air, their way of life hung in the balance.

Led by Chief Red Hawk, the tribe vowed to defend their ancestral lands against the tide of Manifest Destiny. With bows drawn and war cries echoing across the valley, they prepared to face their oppressors with the strength of their ancestors flowing through their veins.

But as the settlers advanced, armed with rifles and cannons, the odds seemed stacked against them. Wave after wave of pioneers surged forward, driven by greed and ambition, heedless of the destruction they left in their wake.

Yet, the Lakota refused to yield. With every arrow loosed and every tomahawk swung, they fought with a ferocity born of desperation. For they knew that to surrender was to consign their children to a life of servitude and suffering.

As the battle raged on, Chief Red Hawk stood tall, his face painted with the symbols of his people's defiance. With a cry that echoed across the plains, he rallied his warriors to one final charge, their spirits unbroken by the ravages of war.

And though the outcome remained uncertain, the Lakota fought on, their courage and resilience serving as a beacon of hope for future generations. For even in the face of overwhelming odds, they refused to let their way of life be extinguished.

10. Stagecoach Showdown

As the stagecoach rumbled through the arid desert, the passengers inside were oblivious to the impending danger lurking nearby. Among them sat a wealthy businessman, a timid schoolteacher, and a retired gunslinger seeking solace in the distant town of Carter.

Suddenly, the coach jolted to a halt, the driver shouting in alarm as masked bandits emerged from the dust, their pistols gleaming in the harsh sunlight. With guns pointed and demands shouted, the passengers were forced to surrender their valuables.

But as the outlaws rifled through their possessions, they failed to notice the schoolteacher slip a small revolver from beneath her petticoats. With nerves of steel, she took aim and fired, catching the leader square in the chest.

Chaos erupted as the bandits scrambled for cover, their carefully laid plans unraveling before their eyes. The retired gunslinger, seizing the opportunity, drew his own weapon and joined the fray, his years of experience evident in every shot fired.

In the midst of the gunfire, the businessman seized his chance, ducking out of the coach and making a run for it, his heart pounding with fear and adrenaline.

Finally, with the bandits driven off and the stagecoach safe once more, the passengers emerged shaken but alive, their unlikely alliance forged in the crucible of danger.

As they continued their journey to Carter, they shared a silent nod of gratitude, knowing that they had faced death together and emerged victorious. In the wild and lawless frontier, sometimes it was the most unexpected events that brought out the true courage of the human spirit.

11. Desert Justice

Under the scorching sun of the Arizona desert, a lone rider cut through the rugged terrain. Dust clouds billowed behind her as she urged her horse onward, her determined eyes fixed on the horizon. But this was no ordinary traveler; this was Kate Morgan, a woman on a mission.

Months ago, her father had been gunned down by a gang of ruthless outlaws. With justice nowhere to be found, Kate took matters into her own hands. Disguised as a man and armed to the teeth, she set out to track down those responsible for her father's death.

As she rode into the sleepy town of Redwood Creek, Kate could feel the tension in the air. The locals eyed her warily, but she paid them no mind. Her focus was on one thing: finding the men who had taken everything from her.

It didn't take long for Kate to pick up the outlaws' trail. They had left a path of destruction in their wake, and she was hot on their heels. With each passing mile, her determination grew stronger, fueled by a burning desire for vengeance.

Finally, she caught up with them at an abandoned mine on the outskirts of town. Without hesitation, Kate sprang into action, guns blazing as she unleashed her fury upon the unsuspecting gang.

When the smoke cleared, the outlaws lay defeated at her feet. Justice had been served, but Kate knew that her journey was far from over. With her father's memory avenged, she rode off into the sunset, a lone figure against the backdrop of the wild frontier.

12. Redemption's Last Stand

The sun dipped low on the horizon, casting long shadows across the dusty streets of Redemption Falls. In the dim light of the saloon, Jim "Six-Shooter" O'Malley nursed a shot of whiskey, the burn of the liquor barely registering against the ache in his chest.

Twenty years he'd been riding, twenty years since he'd hung up his guns for good. But the past has a way of catching up, and tonight, it came knocking at his door.

The swing doors creaked open, and in stepped Cole Thornton, a man Jim hadn't seen since they'd ridden together with the Bar-T outfit. The years had been kinder to Cole; he still had that glint of danger in his eye, while Jim wore his sins like a badge of honor.

"Thought I'd find you here," Cole said, his voice low and dangerous.

Jim tensed, ready for whatever was coming. He'd been expecting this moment, dreading it even, but he'd be damned if he let Cole catch him off guard.

"What do you want, Thornton?" Jim growled, his hand inching towards the Colt at his hip.

Cole leaned against the bar, a smirk playing at the corners of his mouth. "Just here to settle an old debt, Six-Shooter. You and me, one last time."

Jim's heart hammered in his chest as he met Cole's gaze. He knew there was no walking away from this, no escaping the ghosts of his past. With a resigned sigh, he nodded.

"Let's finish it then."

13. Train Robbery Showdown

As the steam engine thundered through the arid desert, its rhythmic chugging echoed against the canyon walls. Inside, passengers huddled nervously, their eyes darting to the windows as the sun dipped low on the horizon.

At the front of the train, a lone figure stood silhouetted against the fading light. Decked in black, with a wide-brimmed hat pulled low over his eyes, he exuded an aura of menace that seemed to fill the entire carriage.

Suddenly, with a deafening blast, the door burst open, and the outlaw leader stepped inside. His eyes gleamed with a mixture of determination and greed as he surveyed the terrified faces before him.

"Listen up, folks," he growled, his voice as sharp as the edge of a knife. "This here's a robbery, and I aim to make it quick and painless."

With swift precision, the outlaw's gang descended upon the passengers, relieving them of their valuables with cold efficiency. Despite their fear, some dared to protest, but a menacing glare from their assailants silenced them instantly.

Meanwhile, outside the train, hidden in the shadows of the desert rocks, a group of lawmen lay in wait. Led by a seasoned marshal, they had been tracking the outlaw gang for months, waiting for the perfect opportunity to strike.

As the robbery reached its climax, the lawmen sprang into action, their guns blazing as they stormed the train. In the chaos that ensued, bullets flew, and shouts filled the air, but when the smoke finally cleared, the outlaw leader lay defeated, justice prevailing in the Wild West once again.

14. Gold and Grit

Amidst the vast expanse of the desert, Jake stumbled upon a glimmer of hope—a nugget of gold peeking out from the sand. His heart raced with excitement as he dug deeper, uncovering a vein of gold that promised unimaginable riches.

But Jake knew the dangers that came with striking gold in these lawless lands. Greedy eyes would be upon him, and he had to tread carefully. He concealed his discovery, working tirelessly to extract the precious metal while keeping a watchful eye for any sign of trouble.

Sure enough, trouble found him soon enough. Bandits prowled the desert, their eyes fixed on Jake's claim. They didn't care about hard work or fair play; they only wanted what they could steal. Jake fortified his camp, setting traps and keeping his trusty revolver close at hand.

As the days passed, tension mounted. Every gust of wind sounded like an approaching enemy, every shadow a potential threat. Yet, Jake refused to give up his claim without a fight. He had poured his blood, sweat, and tears into this land, and he wouldn't let anyone take it from him.

Finally, the bandits struck, launching a relentless assault on Jake's camp. But he was ready, his determination matched only by his skill with a gun. Shots rang out in the desert air as Jake defended what was rightfully his.

When the dust settled, the bandits lay defeated, and Jake stood victorious. He had faced danger from all sides and emerged triumphant, his claim to the gold stronger than ever. And as he surveyed the vast expanse of his land, he knew that no amount of danger could deter him from his dreams of wealth and prosperity.

15. Showdown for Supremacy

In the dust-choked streets of Redwood Gulch, tensions simmered like water in a sun-baked creek bed. The air crackled with anticipation, every creak of a weathered sign, every whistle of the wind, a harbinger of the storm about to break.

At the heart of the turmoil stood Jake Doyle, a lean figure with eyes like flint and a reputation as cold as the iron on his hip. He'd clawed his way up from nothing, building a small fortune on the sweat and blood of others. But now, the walls were closing in.

Across town, the Marshall gang plotted their next move. Led by the ruthless Tom Marshall, they'd long coveted Doyle's turf, and tonight, they aimed to claim it.

As dusk painted the sky with hues of crimson and gold, the two factions met in the shadow of the old mine, the town's lifeblood coursing through its veins like liquid gold.

Words were scarce as gunslingers squared off, their fingers twitching against the polished wood of their weapons. The tension hung heavy in the air, a palpable thing that seemed to weigh down on every soul in the street.

Then, with a thunderous roar, the first shot rang out, setting off a chain reaction that echoed through the canyon like a death knell. Bullets flew, cutting through the air like angry hornets, leaving chaos and destruction in their wake.

In the end, when the smoke cleared and the echoes faded, only one man remained standing. And as he surveyed the wreckage of what was once his kingdom, Jake Doyle knew that the price of power was steep indeed. But in the wild west, survival was its own reward, and he'd be damned if he didn't come out on top.

16. Redemption's Road

Robert Mercer rode alone through the arid dust clouds and scorching sun of the Arizona desert. His reputation preceded him, the whispers of his name echoing in the saloons and among the tumbleweeds. But Robert wasn't the same man he once was.

Years of running had left him tired, haunted by the faces of those he'd wronged. The money he'd amassed through theft and duels meant nothing now; his heart longed for redemption, for a chance to make things right.

He rode into the small town of Salt Furnace, his face hidden beneath the brim of his hat. The wanted posters plastered on the sheriff's office wall had faded, but the bounty on his head remained unchanged.

Despite the risk, Robert found himself drawn to the town's chapel. Inside, he knelt before the altar, his hands clasped in silent prayer. For the first time in years, he spoke to a higher power, seeking forgiveness for the sins he'd committed.

As he left the chapel, Robert stumbled upon a group of bandits terrorizing the townsfolk. Without hesitation, he drew his pistols, his fingers steady and his aim true. In a flurry of gunfire, he dispatched the outlaws, saving the town from certain destruction.

The grateful townsfolk gathered around Robert, their faces filled with awe and admiration. For the first time in years, Robert felt a glimmer of hope. Perhaps redemption was within his reach after all.

With a newfound sense of purpose, Robert vowed to protect the innocent, to make amends for his past transgressions. As he rode out of Salt Furnace, he knew that his journey was far from over, but for the first time in years, he rode with his head held high.

17. Easton Reconciliation

The dusty streets of Easton were silent, save for the creak of the saloon's swinging doors and the distant howl of a coyote. In the heart of town, the tension hung thick like the desert heat, as the Hatfield and McCoy families stood on opposite ends, eyes locked in a fierce standoff.

It started with a dispute over grazing land, but soon, it escalated into a bitter feud that tore the town apart. Each family claimed their right to the land, unwilling to yield an inch to the other. Shootouts became commonplace, and blood stained the sun-baked earth.

Sheriff Sam Collins, a weary man with a badge tarnished by years of futile attempts at peacekeeping, knew the situation was spiraling out of control. He had seen too many lives lost to the feud, too many mothers grieving for their sons.

But on this fateful day, as the tension reached its breaking point, Sheriff Collins made a bold decision. With a voice weathered by years of command, he called for a truce. Surprisingly, both families hesitated, their eyes flickering with uncertainty.

In that moment of hesitation, Sheriff Collins seized the opportunity to broker a ceasefire. He reminded them of the families torn apart, the children left fatherless, and the wives widowed by senseless violence. Slowly, begrudgingly, the Hatfields and McCoys lowered their weapons.

As the sun dipped below the horizon, casting an orange glow over the town, a fragile peace settled over Easton. It was a peace built on the ashes of old grievances, a peace that Sheriff Collins hoped would endure long after the echoes of gunfire had faded into memory.

18. Posse of the Dust

The sun dipped low on the horizon, casting long shadows over the dusty streets of Carter. Sheriff Jake Patterson leaned against the wooden railing of the sheriff's office, his eyes scanning the main thoroughfare for any signs of trouble.

As if on cue, a raucous commotion erupted outside the saloon. Jake sighed and straightened up, knowing he had to intervene before things got out of hand. He stepped out onto the boardwalk, his spurs jingling with each measured stride.

"What's going on here?" he demanded, his voice cutting through the din.

A group of rough-looking cowboys turned to face him, their expressions defiant. "Just minding our own business, Sheriff," one of them replied, his hand resting on the butt of his revolver.

Jake narrowed his eyes, sizing up the men before him. He knew he couldn't handle them alone – not without risking a shootout that would tear his town apart. That's when inspiration struck.

"Listen up, boys," he said, his tone firm but even. "I'm putting together a posse to help keep the peace around here. Anyone interested in earning an honest day's pay and a chance to make a difference, meet me at the jailhouse tomorrow morning."

There was a moment of silence as the cowboys exchanged uncertain glances. Then, one by one, they nodded their agreement and dispersed into the night.

Jake watched them go, a sense of satisfaction swelling in his chest. With a ragtag group of misfits at his side, he knew that together they could bring law and order back to Carter – one dusty street at a time.

19. The Hunter's Stand

Jed rode his weary horse toward the vast plains where the buffalo roamed. His rifle was his only companion, besides the distant echoes of the wild.

For years, Jed had eked out a living hunting buffalo, but now the land was changing. Wealthy landowners sought to claim it for themselves, pushing out the hunters who had lived off the land for generations.

One such landowner, Bartholomew Grimes, was infamous for his greed and cruelty. He had his sights set on the buffalo's grazing grounds, and he wouldn't let anyone stand in his way.

Jed's heart raced as he spotted the herd in the distance. He knew he had to act fast before Grimes' hired guns arrived to drive them off.

With practiced precision, Jed took aim and fired, felling one of the massive beasts with a single shot. But before he could claim his prize, Grimes' men rode in, guns blazing.

Jed fought with all his strength, his bullets finding their mark amidst the chaos. But outnumbered and outgunned, he knew he couldn't hold them off for long.

Just when all seemed lost, a group of fellow hunters arrived, rallying to Jed's side. Together, they drove Grimes' men back, securing the buffalo's freedom for another day.

As the dust settled, Jed knew the fight was far from over. But with his comrades by his side, he was ready to face whatever challenges lay ahead in the ever-changing West.

20. Rebellion's End

In the forgotten stretches of the borderlands a shadowy figure rode into view. It was Ramón Alvarez, a notorious bandit with a vendetta against the American settlers encroaching on his homeland.

Gripping his pistol tightly, Ramón spurred his horse onward, his eyes ablaze with determination. Behind him, a ragtag group of rebels followed, their faces hardened by years of oppression.

Their destination: a small settlement nestled amidst the rugged terrain. Ramón's heart pounded with anticipation as they approached, his mind filled with memories of the injustices suffered at the hands of the settlers.

As they neared the outskirts of the town, Ramón signaled for his men to halt. With a nod, they fanned out, ready to strike at a moment's notice. Ramón dismounted, his boots kicking up dust as he strode forward.

The settlers emerged from their homes, their expressions wary as they eyed the approaching bandits. Ramón stepped forward, his voice ringing out with authority.

"We demand justice for our people!" he declared, his words echoing through the dusty streets. "You have taken our land, our livelihoods. Now, we will take back what is rightfully ours!"

Tension hung thick in the air as the settlers faced off against the rebels. But before violence could erupt, a voice rang out from the crowd.

"Stop this madness!" It was María, a young woman who had grown up alongside Ramón. Her eyes pleaded for peace, her words a plea for reason.

Ramón hesitated, his gaze softening as he met María's eyes. In that moment, he saw the futility of their vendetta, the endless cycle of bloodshed and loss.

With a heavy heart, Ramón lowered his weapon, signaling an end to the rebellion. As the sun dipped below the horizon, casting long shadows across the desert, Ramón vowed to forge a new path—one of peace and reconciliation.

21. Echoes of Vengeance

Alone under the vast expanse of the western sky, Cole Harris rode through the desolate plains. His face bore the scars of loss, etched deep by the brutal attack that had claimed his family and his home. Determination set his jaw as he pursued his only purpose now: vengeance.

The smoke of his burning homestead still hung in the air as he rode toward the distant mountains, where the renegade Indian tribe was said to dwell. Each step of his horse stirred the dust of his past, fueling the fire of his fury.

Days turned into weeks as Cole tracked the elusive tribe, surviving on nothing but his will and the unyielding thirst for retribution. When he finally found them, his heart pounded like the thunder of a distant storm. His hand tightened around the grip of his Colt revolver, its cold steel a comfort against the searing heat of his rage.

Under the cover of night, Cole crept into their camp, his shadow blending with the darkness. With the stealth of a desert fox, he closed in on his prey, his breath a silent prayer for the justice he sought.

But as he stood over the sleeping forms of his enemies, his hand stayed, frozen by a flicker of doubt. In their faces, he saw not the savages he had imagined, but men like himself, driven by their own tragedies and their own quest for survival.

With a heavy heart, Cole lowered his gun. Revenge, he realized, was a hollow victory. Turning his back on the camp, he rode into the dawn, leaving behind the ghosts of his past and embracing the promise of a new beginning.

22. Shadows of Tombstone

The sun dipped low on the horizon, casting long shadows across the streets of Tombstone. The townsfolk whispered in hushed tones as they gathered at the saloon, seeking refuge from the growing fear that gripped their hearts.

Sheriff Ray Walker stood tall in the center of the room, his eyes scanning the crowd with a mix of determination and concern. For weeks now, Tombstone had been plagued by a series of gruesome killings, each one more brutal than the last.

No one knew who – or what – was behind the murders. Some said it was the work of a vengeful spirit, while others whispered of a bloodthirsty outlaw seeking revenge. But one thing was certain: the killer had to be stopped before more lives were lost.

As the night wore on, tension hung heavy in the air, suffocating the once lively atmosphere of the saloon. Sheriff Walker knew he had to act fast if he was to restore peace to Tombstone.

With a steely resolve, he rallied a group of brave volunteers to join him in hunting down the elusive killer. Together, they combed the desolate plains surrounding the town, following any lead that might bring them closer to their quarry.

Days turned into weeks, and still, the killer remained one step ahead of them. But Sheriff Walker refused to give up hope, knowing that the fate of Tombstone rested in his hands.

And then, one fateful night, they stumbled upon a hidden cave deep in the heart of the wilderness. Inside, they found the killer lurking in the shadows, his eyes gleaming with malice.

With guns drawn and hearts pounding, Sheriff Walker and his posse prepared for the final showdown. It was time to bring justice to Tombstone, no matter the cost.

23. The Last Ride of Butch Cassidy

Born Robert Leroy Parker in Utah in 1866, Butch Cassidy was drawn to a life of crime from a young age. With a quick wit and a silver tongue, he soon became known as one of the most notorious bank and train robbers in the West, leading a band of outlaws known as the "Wild Bunch."

But it was not just his skill with a gun that made Butch Cassidy a legend—it was his charm and charisma, his ability to elude capture time and time again, and his unwavering loyalty to his friends and comrades.

In 1901, after years on the run from the law, Butch Cassidy and his partner, the Sundance Kid, fled to South America in search of a new beginning. There, they continued their life of crime, robbing banks and stagecoaches across the continent with impunity.

But the end was drawing near. In 1908, Butch Cassidy and the Sundance Kid were cornered by Bolivian soldiers in a remote village in the Andes Mountains.

Surrounded and outnumbered, they fought bravely to the bitter end, choosing death over capture.

And so, the legend of Butch Cassidy came to an end—a tale of adventure, romance, and rebellion that would live on in American folklore - the enduring allure of the outlaw hero.

24. Riding Against the Odds

Under the unforgiving Texan sun, Clara Jensen tightened her grip on the reins as she rode across the vast expanse of her family's ranch. With her father's recent passing, the responsibility of running the ranch now fell squarely on her shoulders. But in a world where men ruled the land, Clara knew she would have to fight twice as hard to prove herself.

Her determination was put to the test when she discovered that rustlers had been stealing cattle from their herd. With no time to waste, Clara gathered her courage and set out to track down the thieves herself. Armed with her father's old Winchester rifle and a steely resolve, she rode out into the rugged terrain, her heart pounding with each passing mile.

As the sun dipped below the horizon, Clara spotted a flickering campfire in the distance. Drawing closer, she found herself face to face with the rustlers, a group of rough-looking men who sneered at her audacity.

Undeterred, Clara leveled her rifle and demanded they return what they had stolen. A tense standoff ensued, but Clara refused to back down. With nerves of steel, she held her ground until the rustlers finally relented, returning the stolen cattle and fleeing into the night.

Returning triumphantly to the ranch, Clara was met with admiration and respect from the ranch hands who had doubted her abilities. Though the road ahead would be challenging, Clara knew that she had proven herself as a capable rancher, ready to carry on her father's legacy in a world that had underestimated her.

25. Desert Redemption

The sun sank low on the horizon, casting long shadows across the barren landscape. Dust billowed from the hooves of a lone horse galloping across the arid plains. Its rider slumped in the saddle, blood staining his shirt, his breaths ragged with pain.

Miranda stood on the porch of her modest cabin, a weary expression etched on her face as she watched the approaching figure. She gripped the shotgun tightly, unsure whether to trust the stranger or fear him. But as he drew nearer, she saw the desperation etched on his face, the way he clutched at his side as if trying to hold himself together.

"Please," he gasped, his voice barely a whisper. "I need help."

She hesitated for only a moment before lowering the gun and stepping forward to offer assistance. With trembling hands, she helped the wounded man down from his horse and guided him inside.

For days, Miranda nursed him back to health, cleaning his wounds and listening to his tales of life on the run. Despite the danger he brought with him, she found herself drawn to his quiet strength and the sadness that lurked behind his eyes.

As the weeks passed, they forged an unlikely bond, two souls brought together by circumstance and a shared longing for redemption. And when the time came for him to leave, Miranda watched him ride off into the sunset, knowing that he would always hold a piece of her heart.

26. Trails of Hope

The wagon wheels creaked and groaned as they rolled across the rugged terrain, the sun beating down on the weary travelers. Among them, Sarah clutched her son tightly, her eyes scanning the horizon for any sign of respite.

Their supplies dwindled, their spirits faltered, but still, they pressed on, driven by the promise of a new beginning in the untouched wilderness. Yet as they journeyed deeper into the unknown, they faced challenges that tested their resolve.

Rivers swelled with treacherous currents, threatening to sweep away their hopes and dreams. Wild animals lurked in the shadows, hungry for the taste of human flesh. And with each passing day, the harsh reality of their situation became painfully clear.

But amid the adversity, a sense of camaraderie emerged among the pioneers. They banded together, supporting one another through the darkest of times. Together, they built makeshift shelters, hunted for food, and defended themselves against the dangers that lurked in the wild.

And when the storms raged and the winds howled, they found solace in each other's company, drawing strength from their shared determination to survive.

As the days turned into weeks and the weeks into months, they carved out a new life in the untamed wilderness. Though they faced hardships and heartaches along the way, they emerged stronger, united by a bond forged in the fires of adversity.

And as they stood atop a windswept hill, gazing out at the vast expanse of land before them, they knew that they had found a home in the unforgiving frontier.

27. A Sheriff's Resolve

In the dim light of dawn, Sheriff Porter rode out from the town of Doan's Crossing, his breath forming icy clouds in the bitter winter air. A series of cattle thefts had plagued the ranchers, and Porter swore to put an end to it.

Following a set of faint tracks, Porter led his horse through the frost-covered plains. The trail twisted and turned, disappearing into thickets and reappearing on frozen creeks. Hours passed, but Porter pressed on, fueled by determination and duty.

As the sun began its descent, Porter spotted smoke rising in the distance. Urging his horse forward, he approached cautiously. Hidden in a small valley, he found the rustlers' camp, surrounded by stolen cattle.

With a quick hand signal, Porter summoned his deputies, and together they descended upon the camp. Shots rang out as the rustlers fought back, but Porter's men held firm, driving the thieves into retreat.

In the aftermath, Porter surveyed the scene, the stolen cattle returned to their rightful owners. Though weary from the battle, a sense of justice warmed his heart. The town of Doan's Crossing would sleep easier tonight, knowing their sheriff had protected their livelihoods.

As the stars blinked to life in the darkening sky, Porter rode back to town, his mission accomplished. Though the winter winds howled around him, he felt a sense of satisfaction knowing that law and order still held sway in the wild frontier.

28. Harmony in Clearwater

In the gentle warmth of a spring morning, Kelsey Dawson rode into the bustling town of Clearwater. As he tethered his horse outside the saloon, he noticed the vibrant energy that filled the air. People bustled about, eager to enjoy the burgeoning life that the season brought.

Inside the saloon, Kelsey sensed an air of tension. Men gathered in hushed clusters, their faces grave as they discussed the latest news. It didn't take long for Kelsey to learn the cause of their concern – a simmering conflict between the sheepherders and the cattlemen, each vying for control of the land.

With a sense of duty stirring within him, Kelsey decided to intervene. He knew all too well the destructive force that unchecked animosity could unleash. Approaching the ranchers and the herders, he offered his services as a mediator, hoping to find a peaceful resolution to their dispute.

At first, his proposition was met with skepticism. What could a drifter possibly know about their way of life? But Kelsey's calm demeanor and unwavering resolve soon won them over, and they reluctantly agreed to give him a chance.

Day by day, Kelsey worked tirelessly to bridge the gap between the two factions, finding common ground where none seemed to exist. With each passing conversation, tensions eased, and mutual understanding began to blossom.

Finally, on a crisp spring evening, the people of Clearwater gathered together in the town square. With Kelsey standing at the forefront, they declared an end to the feud that had threatened to tear their community apart.

As the sun dipped below the horizon, casting a warm glow over the town, Kelsey couldn't help but smile. In a world where conflict was all too common, he had helped bring about a rare moment of peace and harmony. And for that, he knew, Clearwater would be forever grateful.

29. The Siege of Dry Creek

The dusty streets of Dry Creek were usually quiet, but on this day, they were filled with fear. A gang of ruthless bank robbers had descended upon the town, leaving chaos and destruction in their wake.

Sheriff Jake Thornton stood tall, his jaw set with determination as he surveyed the scene. The outlaws had barricaded themselves inside the bank, holding hostages and daring anyone to challenge them.

With no time to waste, Jake rallied a group of brave townsfolk to help him confront the criminals. They armed themselves with whatever they could find, ready to stand up to the invaders and protect their home.

As they approached the bank, gunfire erupted, filling the air with smoke and screams. Jake's heart raced as he led the charge, bullets whizzing past him as he took cover behind a wagon.

With nerves of steel, Jake and his makeshift posse fought tooth and nail against the outlaws, inching closer to the bank with each passing moment. They knew that failure was not an option – the lives of their friends and neighbors depended on their success.

After a fierce battle that seemed to last an eternity, the outlaws finally surrendered, their leader taken down by Jake's precise aim. As the dust settled, the townsfolk breathed a collective sigh of relief, grateful for their sheriff's bravery and unwavering resolve.

In the days that followed, Dry Creek began to heal from the scars of the siege. The townsfolk held their heads a little higher, knowing that they had faced adversity together and emerged stronger than ever. And Sheriff Jake Thornton remained a symbol of hope and courage in the wild frontier.

30. Freedom's Frontier

Tucker's boots crunched on the dusty path, each step a testament to the miles he'd traveled. The sun beat down relentlessly, but he welcomed its warmth after the bitter cold of his past.

Born into servitude, Tucker had known little of freedom until he took up the gun. Now, he rode west, chasing whispers of opportunity and liberty.

His journey led him to a small town nestled in the heart of the prairie, where the promise of a fresh start beckoned. But freedom wasn't easy to come by, not for a man like him.

In the saloon, eyes followed him warily as he entered, their gazes filled with suspicion and prejudice. But Tucker paid them no mind. He'd seen worse in his time.

He found work as a ranch hand, earning his keep with sweat and toil. But even as he built a life for himself, the shadows of his past loomed large.

When trouble came to town in the form of a ruthless gang, Tucker didn't hesitate to stand against them. With his guns blazing, he fought for the freedom he'd long sought.

In the end, it wasn't just about surviving—it was about reclaiming his dignity and his right to live on his own terms.

As the dust settled and the last of the outlaws lay defeated, Tucker stood tall, his spirit unbroken. For in the West, where the horizon stretched wide and the sky knew no bounds, there was always room for a man to make his mark. And Tucker intended to do just that.

31. Where the Wind Carries Hope

Jeb Brown rode hard across the Arizona desert, his eyes squinting against the glare as he searched the horizon. His brother, Will, had vanished three days ago, leaving only a cryptic note behind. Determined to uncover the truth, Jeb followed the sparse trail, his heart heavy with worry.

As he rode deeper into the rugged landscape, Jeb's thoughts drifted to their childhood days spent on their father's ranch. Will had always been the reckless one, chasing adventure while Jeb toiled in the fields. But blood was thicker than water, and Jeb would move mountains to find his brother.

As dusk settled over the land, Jeb made camp by a solitary mesquite tree, the flickering flames of his campfire casting eerie shadows on the surrounding rocks. The desert was a harsh mistress, unforgiving to those who dared to tread her sands alone.

The next morning, Jeb's quest led him to the ramshackle town of Helena, a haven for drifters and outcasts. Here, he hoped to find answers amidst the tumbleweeds and saloons that lined the dusty streets.

His inquiries soon caught the attention of a grizzled old prospector who claimed to have seen Will heading west towards the mountains. With renewed determination, Jeb set off once more, his horse's hooves pounding a steady rhythm against the hard-packed earth.

As the sun dipped low in the sky, Jeb finally caught sight of a figure silhouetted against the fading light. It was Will, battered and bruised but alive. With tears of relief in his eyes, Jeb spurred his horse forward, ready to bring his brother home.

32. A Pinkerton's Pursuit

The town of Redwood Creek was abuzz with whispers of the latest train robbery. As the sun dipped behind the rugged mountains, a lone figure rode into town, dust swirling in his wake. Marshal John Hayes, a Pinkerton detective, dismounted in front of the sheriff's office.

Inside, Sheriff McCall greeted him with a grim expression. "Another one, John. This time, they hit the express train heading west. Cleaned it out like they knew every move."

John's eyes narrowed. He'd been tracking this gang for months, and they always seemed one step ahead. "Any witnesses?"

The sheriff shook his head. "Not a soul. They're like ghosts."

John clenched his jaw, his resolve hardening. He knew he had to act fast before more innocent lives were endangered.

The next morning, John saddled his horse and set out to investigate the scene of the crime. He combed through the wreckage, searching for any clue that might lead him to the perpetrators.

Hours passed, the sun climbing higher in the sky, but John remained undeterred. Finally, he spotted a faint set of tracks leading away from the scene.

Following them deep into the wilderness, John's senses sharpened. He knew he was getting closer.

At last, he stumbled upon a hidden camp nestled in a secluded canyon. The outlaws were caught off guard as John burst into their midst, guns drawn.

A fierce gunfight ensued, bullets whizzing through the air as John faced the notorious bandit leader. In the end, justice prevailed, and John emerged victorious.

As he rode back into town with the gang in tow, the townsfolk cheered his name. Another victory for law and order in the wild west.

33. Whispers of Deadwood

Amidst the desolate sands of the Mojave Desert lay the forgotten town of Deadwood. Its abandoned buildings whispered tales of gold rushes and lost dreams. Dust devils danced in the ghostly streets as the sun dipped low on the horizon.

Nash, a weathered gunslinger with a past as mysterious as the desert itself, stumbled upon Deadwood by chance. Seeking shelter from an approaching sandstorm, he took refuge in what appeared to be an old saloon.

Inside, he found more than just shelter. A faded map, half-buried beneath layers of dust, caught his eye. With trembling hands, he brushed off the debris to reveal the promise of hidden treasure.

The map led him through the maze of abandoned buildings, past crumbling facades and forgotten memories. Each step brought him closer to the heart of Deadwood, where legend whispered of untold riches.

As the moon rose high in the sky, casting an eerie glow over the deserted town, Nash finally reached his destination. Beneath the floorboards of the old bank, he unearthed a chest filled with glittering gold and precious gems.

But his triumph was short-lived. The sound of approaching hoofbeats shattered the silence of the night. Outlaws, drawn by the promise of wealth, descended upon Deadwood like vultures to carrion.

With bullets flying and shadows dancing in the moonlight, Nash fought to protect his newfound treasure. In the chaos that followed, he realized that some treasures were better left buried in the sands of time.

34. Desert Reckoning

The sun beat down mercilessly on the arid plains as Laura leaned against the weathered fence, surveying the vast expanse of her family's ranch. Dust swirled in the hot breeze, carrying with it the scent of parched earth and desperation.

For generations, the Johnson ranch had been a beacon of hope in the unforgiving landscape of the West. But now, faced with mounting debts and relentless pressure from the bank, Laura's dreams were slipping away like grains of sand through her fingers.

With steely determination, she refused to surrender. Each morning before dawn, she saddled her horse and rode out to check on the herd, her mind racing with plans to save her family's legacy.

But time was running out. The bank's threats grew more ominous with each passing day, and Laura knew she needed a miracle to turn the tide in her favor.

One evening, as the sun dipped below the horizon, casting the sky in hues of fiery orange and crimson, Laura received an unexpected visitor. It was an old friend, a fellow rancher who had weathered his fair share of hardships.

With a knowing glint in his eye, he offered Laura a lifeline – a chance to join forces with him and several other struggling ranchers to fight back against the tyranny of the banks.

With renewed hope coursing through her veins, Laura agreed. Together, they rallied their fellow ranchers, organizing protests and petitions to demand fair treatment from the banks.

And as the dust settled and the sun set on the horizon, Laura stood tall, her family's ranch saved from the brink of disaster, a testament to the power of resilience and community in the Wild West.

35. Kit Carson

Kit Carson was a frontiersman, scout, and legend whose exploits would capture the imagination of generations to come.

Born in the wilderness of Kentucky in 1809, Kit Carson was drawn to a life of adventure from a young age. As a teenager, he left home to seek his fortune in the vast expanses of the West, finding work as a trapper, hunter, and guide for fur-trading expeditions.

But it was as a scout and explorer that Kit Carson truly made his mark. With his intimate knowledge of the land and his fearless spirit, he blazed trails through some of the most untamed wilderness in America, from the Rocky Mountains to the deserts of the Southwest.

In 1842, Carson joined the famous Fremont Expedition, embarking on a series of daring journeys that would take him deep into uncharted territory. From mapping the Oregon Trail to exploring the Great Basin and the Sierra Nevada, Carson's exploits captured the attention of the nation and solidified his reputation as one of the greatest explorers of his time.

But it was his role in the conquest of the West that would secure his place in history. As a scout for the U.S. Army during the Mexican-American War and the Indian Wars that followed, Carson played a pivotal role in shaping the destiny of the American West, guiding settlers, soldiers, and wagon trains through the treacherous wilderness and helping to secure the frontier for future generations.

And though his life was filled with danger and hardship, Kit Carson never wavered in his commitment to exploration and adventure. For him, the call of the wild was a siren song that could never be ignored.

36. The Outlaw's Reckoning

The rugged streets of Copper Canyon were quiet as the sun began its descent behind the towering cliffs. In the fading light, a group of shadowy figures emerged from the outskirts, their faces hidden beneath the brims of their hats.

Among them was Chet Cole, a notorious outlaw known for his quick draw and ruthless tactics. He had gathered his gang, vowing revenge on Sheriff Dawson, the man responsible for their imprisonment.

They rode into town under the cover of darkness, their horses' hooves echoing against the wooden planks of the deserted streets. The saloons and shops were closed, the townsfolk holed up in their homes, oblivious to the danger outside.

As they reached the sheriff's office, Chet dismounted and strode towards the door, his six-shooter glinting in the moonlight. With a swift kick, he sent the door crashing open, revealing Sheriff Dawson seated at his desk, cleaning his gun.

The sheriff's eyes widened in surprise as Chet leveled his pistol at him, a menacing grin spreading across his face. "Remember me, Sheriff?" he sneered. "I'm here to settle the score."

But before he could pull the trigger, a gunshot pierced the air from the shadows, striking Chet in the shoulder and sending him sprawling to the ground. The other outlaws scattered, vanishing into the night as the sheriff's deputies emerged from hiding, guns drawn.

Sheriff Dawson approached Chet, his expression solemn. "Looks like justice caught up with you, Cole," he said, holstering his weapon. "You and your gang are going back where you belong: behind bars."

As the last of the outlaws was led away, the sheriff turned back to his office, knowing that the fight for law and order in Copper Canyon was far from over.

37. Iron Frontier

In the rugged terrain of the Sierra Nevada mountains, where the land seemed to defy human effort, Liang Chen, a Chinese immigrant, saw opportunity. With a dream as vast as the open sky, he set out to build a railroad that would connect the coast to the heart of the country.

Despite the skepticism of many, Liang was undeterred. Armed with little more than determination and grit, he rallied a team of fellow immigrants and began the arduous task of laying tracks through the unforgiving landscape.

Days turned into weeks, and weeks into months, as the workers toiled under the scorching sun and biting cold of the mountains. But Liang's vision never wavered, and inch by inch, the railroad began to take shape.

Yet, as progress was made, so too came challenges. The land fought back with landslides and rockslides, threatening to undo all their hard work. But Liang refused to be defeated, leading his team with unwavering resolve.

Finally, after years of tireless effort, the railroad was complete. The first train chugged triumphantly across the tracks, heralding a new era of prosperity for the region.

But for Liang, the journey was far from over. As the railroad brought prosperity, it also brought prejudice and hostility towards the Chinese immigrants who had built it. Undeterred, Liang continued to fight for acceptance and equality, determined to leave a legacy that would endure long after the last train had passed.

In the shadow of the Sierra Nevada mountains, Liang Chen's railroad stood as a tribute to the power of perseverance and the enduring spirit of those who dared to dream.

38. Whispers of Victory

In the dimly lit saloon of Whispering Pines, the clinking of glasses and murmurs of conversation filled the air. At a corner table, a group of rugged men gathered around a worn poker table, their eyes fixed on the young gunslinger seated among them.

Jake Baxter, known for his lightning-fast draw and sharp wit, had come to Whispering Pines to make a name for himself. And what better way to do it than by winning big in a high-stakes poker game?

As the cards were dealt, tension hung heavy in the air. The stakes were high, and the players knew it. Each hand was played with precision, the pot growing with every round.

Jake remained calm and focused, his mind calculating every move. He had studied the game for years, honing his skills in back-alley games and seedy saloons. Now, it was time to put those skills to the test.

With each hand, Jake's confidence grew. He bluffed and raised, his opponents falling one by one to his cunning strategy. The pile of chips in front of him grew steadily, a testament to his skill and nerve.

But just when victory seemed within his grasp, a newcomer entered the saloon. A notorious gunslinger known as Swift Hawkins, his reputation preceded him. With a cocky grin, he sauntered over to the table, eager to join the game.

The atmosphere grew tense as the final hand was dealt. Jake and Swift faced off, their eyes locked in a silent battle of wills. And as the cards were revealed, Jake's heart pounded in his chest.

In the end, it was Jake who emerged victorious, his name now etched in the annals of Whispering Pines' history as the gunslinger who bested Swift Hawkins in a game of poker.

39. Border Justice

In the rugged terrain of the Texas-Mexico border, dust clouds swirled as the relentless sun beat down on the barren landscape. Texas Ranger Grant Westbrook spurred his horse forward, his eyes fixed on the distant horizon where a gang of outlaws had disappeared with stolen cattle.

With his trusted revolver holstered at his side, Grant rode hard, his determination unwavering despite the scorching heat. The tracks of the outlaws were faint, but Grant's instincts guided him, leading him deeper into the unforgiving wilderness.

As the sun dipped low on the horizon, Grant finally spotted the flicker of a campfire in the distance. Drawing closer, he saw the outlaws lounging around the fire, their faces obscured by the shadows of the night.

Grant dismounted quietly, his movements stealthy as he crept closer to the camp. With a swift and silent approach, he positioned himself behind a large boulder, his hand hovering over his revolver.

With a sudden burst of movement, Grant emerged from his hiding spot, his gun drawn and aimed squarely at the outlaws. "Texas Ranger!" he bellowed, his voice echoing through the still night air.

The outlaws sprang to their feet, reaching for their own weapons, but Grant was faster. With lightning speed, he fired off a volley of shots, each one finding its mark with deadly accuracy.

In the aftermath of the shootout, Grant stood alone amidst the fallen outlaws, his breath coming in ragged gasps. Though the battle was won, Grant knew that his work was far from over. With a steely resolve, he mounted his horse and continued his pursuit into the wild unknown.

40. Tattered Flags

The war had ended, but for Jedediah Monroe, the battle raged on within. Once a proud Confederate soldier, he returned home to the dusty plains of Texas a changed man. The air was thick with the scent of gunpowder and the memories of fallen comrades.

Haunted by the horrors he had witnessed on the battlefield, Jedediah struggled to find his place in a world torn apart by conflict. The once bustling town of Cedar Creek had become a mere shadow of its former self, its streets deserted and its buildings crumbling.

As Jedediah wandered through the desolate town, he couldn't help but feel a sense of emptiness gnawing at his soul. His family's farm lay in ruins, its fields barren and its fences broken. The war had taken everything from him, leaving him with nothing but the bitter taste of defeat.

But just when all hope seemed lost, Jedediah found solace in an unexpected place. It was in the company of Sarah Carter, a widow who had lost her husband to the war. Together, they found comfort in each other's arms, their shared grief forging a bond that transcended the pain of the past.

With Sarah's love and support, Jedediah began to rebuild his life, brick by brick. He traded his rifle for a plow, tilling the soil and sowing the seeds of a new beginning. Though the scars of war would never fully heal, Jedediah found peace in knowing that he was not alone in his struggle.

And as the sun set on the horizon, casting its golden glow over the Texas plains, Jedediah knew that he had finally found his place in the world. For in the quiet embrace of Cedar Creek, he had discovered that even in the darkest of times, there is still light to be found.

41. Redemption's Resolve

In the rugged expanse of the New Mexico Territory, where the heat dried the earth and grit choked the air, stood a lone figure with a past as dark as the night sky above. His name was Caleb Morgan, once feared as the deadliest gunfighter in the West. But now, he sought redemption for the lives he had taken.

When word reached Caleb of a bandit gang terrorizing a group of settlers making their way westward, he knew he had to act. For too long, he had wandered aimlessly, haunted by the ghosts of his past. This was his chance to make amends, to atone for his sins and find peace at last.

With steely determination, Caleb rode out to meet the settlers, his Colt Peacemaker strapped to his hip. He found them huddled together in a makeshift camp, their faces etched with fear and uncertainty. They were no match for the ruthless outlaws who preyed upon the weak and defenseless.

But Caleb was not about to let them fall victim to such lawlessness. Drawing upon his years of experience, he trained the settlers in the art of self-defense, teaching them to shoot and ride like true frontier folk. Together, they stood united against the coming storm.

When the bandits finally arrived, they were met with a fierce resistance they had not anticipated. Bullets flew and blood was spilled, but Caleb and the settlers held their ground, their resolve unbroken. In the end, justice prevailed, and the bandits were driven off into the desert.

As the dust settled and the sun dipped below the horizon, Caleb looked upon the settlers with a sense of pride. He may never be able to erase the sins of his past, but in protecting the innocent, he had found a measure of redemption. And for that, he was grateful.

42. Trailblazing Jane

Over in the sprawling plains of the Dakota Territory, where the grass stretched endlessly and the sky seemed to touch the horizon, there was a young woman named Jane who longed for adventure beyond the confines of her father's ranch.

Despite her father's objections, Jane was determined to prove herself as capable as any man. So, when the opportunity arose to join a cattle drive bound for the Kansas railhead, she saw her chance to break free from the constraints of society.

Disguised as a boy named Jack, Jane slipped away in the dead of night, leaving behind the safety of her home to pursue her dreams of the open range. She rode with the cowboys, her heart pounding with excitement as they herded the cattle across the rugged terrain.

But life on the trail was not easy for Jane. She faced harsh weather, stampedes, and the constant threat of danger from outlaws and wild animals. Yet, she refused to falter, determined to prove herself worthy of her place among the men.

As the days turned into weeks and the miles stretched on, Jane earned the respect of her fellow cowboys with her grit and determination. She roped and rode with the best of them, her true identity hidden beneath layers of dirt and sweat.

But it wasn't until disaster struck in the form of a raging prairie fire that Jane's true bravery was put to the test. With flames licking at their heels and the cattle in a panic, she led the drive to safety, risking life and limb to ensure their survival.

When the smoke cleared and the danger had passed, Jane emerged from the ashes a hero in the eyes of her comrades. No longer just a girl playing dress-up, but a trailblazer in her own right, proving that courage knows no gender on the unforgiving frontier.

43. Shadows of Justice

Deputy Marshal Sam Travis patrolled the dusty streets of Goodwill with a watchful eye, his hand never straying far from the grip of his Colt revolver. As the right-hand man to Sheriff Hank Dawson, Sam took his duty to uphold the law seriously, even when the odds were stacked against him.

One hot afternoon, while making his rounds on the outskirts of town, Sam stumbled upon a group of men huddled in whispered conversation near the edge of the farmers' fields. Suspicious of their clandestine meeting, he concealed himself behind a stand of mesquite bushes and listened intently to their conversation.

To his dismay, Sam soon discovered that the men were part of a sinister plot to cheat the local farmers out of their land. Led by the corrupt land baron, Horace Beacher, they planned to use intimidation and violence to force the farmers off their homesteads, paving the way for Beacher to seize control of the land for himself.

With the future of Goodwill hanging in the balance, Sam knew he couldn't turn a blind eye to the injustice unfolding before him. Despite the risks, he resolved to confront Beacher and his cronies head-on, determined to protect the hardworking men and women who called the town home.

Armed with nothing but his wits and his iron will, Sam waged a one-man crusade against the forces of greed and corruption that threatened to tear the community apart. With each step he took, he drew closer to uncovering the truth behind Beacher's scheme and bringing the perpetrators to justice.

In the end, it was Sam's unwavering determination and unyielding sense of duty that saved Goodwill from ruin. Though the road was long and fraught with danger, he stood tall as a beacon of hope in the face of darkness, proving that even the smallest of men can cast the longest shadows of justice.

44. Trails of Destiny

Amid the towering peaks of the Rocky Mountains, where the air was thin and the silence deafening, lived a solitary figure known only as the Mountain Man. He was a rugged soul, weathered by years spent traversing the untamed wilderness, and his knowledge of the land was unmatched by any who dared to challenge it.

When a group of settlers arrived in the nearby town of Whispering Pines, seeking passage to the fertile lands beyond the mountains, they turned to the Mountain Man for guidance. Though reluctant at first to take on the responsibility, he ultimately agreed to lead them through the treacherous terrain, knowing that the journey would be fraught with peril at every turn.

With their wagons loaded with supplies and their spirits high, the settlers set out into the unknown under the Mountain Man's watchful eye. For weeks they forged ahead, following winding trails and crossing rushing rivers, their determination unwavering in the face of adversity.

But as they ventured deeper into the heart of the mountains, they encountered challenges they could never have imagined. Fierce storms battered their camp, wolves howled in the night, and supplies dwindled with each passing day. Yet through it all, the Mountain Man remained a steady presence, guiding them with quiet strength and unwavering resolve.

As they neared their destination, the settlers looked to the Mountain Man with newfound respect and gratitude. Though he was a man of few words, his actions spoke volumes, and they knew that they owed their survival to his expertise and courage.

In the end, as they stood on the threshold of their new home, the settlers bid farewell to the Mountain Man with heavy hearts, knowing that they owed him a debt that could never be repaid. And as he disappeared into the wilderness once more, they whispered a silent prayer of thanks to the man who had led them safely through the trails of destiny.

45. Shadows on the Range

In the vast expanse of the open range, where the weather never relented and the wind whispered secrets across the dusty plains, lived a rancher named Jeb Turner. He was a proud man, with weathered hands and a heart as tough as the land he called home.

One fateful morning, Jeb awoke to find that his prized herd of cattle had vanished without a trace. Anger burned in his veins as he surveyed the empty fields, knowing that the loss would spell ruin for his struggling ranch. Determined to recover what was rightfully his, Jeb set out to find the thieves responsible.

With few leads to go on, Jeb turned to the only man he knew could help him: a gunslinger by the name of Luke Cassidy. Known for his sharp wit and even sharper aim, Luke was a force to be reckoned with on the open range, and Jeb knew that he would stop at nothing to track down the stolen cattle.

Together, Jeb and Luke embarked on a perilous journey across the rugged terrain, following the faintest traces of hoofprints and whispers of rumors. Along the way, they encountered danger at every turn, from vicious outlaws to unforgiving elements. Yet through it all, their determination never wavered, fueled by the promise of justice and the hope of reclaiming what had been lost.

As they closed in on their quarry, tensions ran high and the stakes grew ever higher. But with their wits and their guns at the ready, Jeb and Luke stood firm against the forces arrayed against them, knowing that victory was within their grasp.

In the end, as the stolen cattle were driven back to the ranch in triumph, Jeb and Luke shared a silent nod of respect, knowing that their bond had been forged in the crucible of the frontier. And as they rode off into the sunset together, shadows lengthening behind them, they knew that they had earned their place among the legends of the open range.

46. Blood of the Ancestors

The echoes of ancient spirits lingered in the whispering winds in the heart of the untamed wilderness where lived a warrior named Wovoka. He was one of the last of his tribe, a proud descendant of those who had roamed the land since time immemorial.

But one fateful day, as the sun dipped low on the horizon and cast long shadows across the land, tragedy struck. A band of ruthless soldiers descended upon Wovoka's village, their guns blazing and their hearts filled with hate. In a merciless onslaught, they slaughtered Wovoka's kin, leaving nothing but death and devastation in their wake.

With the blood of his people staining the earth and the cries of the fallen echoing in his ears, Wovoka swore an oath of vengeance upon the invaders who had stolen everything from him. With his bow in hand and his spirit unbroken, he set out into the wilderness, determined to track down those responsible and make them pay for their crimes.

For days and nights without end, Wovoka stalked his prey with the skill and cunning of a predator on the hunt. Along the way, he encountered allies and adversaries alike, each one proof to the harsh realities of life on the frontier.

But through it all, Wovoka remained steadfast in his quest, driven by a burning desire for justice and a thirst for retribution. And when he finally confronted the English soldiers who had wrought such devastation upon his people, he met them with the fury of a storm unleashed, his arrows finding their marks with deadly precision.

In the end, as the last of his enemies lay vanquished at his feet, Wovoka stood alone amidst the wreckage of his once-proud village. But though the scars of the past would never fully heal, he knew that his people's memory would live on in the land itself, forever enshrined in the blood of the ancestors.

47. Shadows Over Sundown

In the sprawling expanse of the Wild West, where lawlessness reigned supreme and justice was but a distant dream, lay the humble town of Sundown. Nestled amidst the rolling hills and dusty plains, it was a place where weary travelers sought refuge from the harsh realities of life on the frontier.

But Sundown was not immune to the shadows that lurked in the darkness, for it harbored a dark secret—a gang of outlaws led by a ruthless gunslinger known only as "The Reaper." With his band of cutthroats at his side, The Reaper struck fear into the hearts of the townsfolk, leaving a trail of blood and destruction in his wake.

For years, the people of Sundown lived in constant fear of The Reaper's reign of terror, their once-peaceful streets now haunted by the specter of violence and lawlessness. But amidst the chaos, there arose a flicker of hope—a lone gunslinger named Luke Carson, determined to bring justice to Sundown and put an end to The Reaper's tyranny once and for all.

With his trusty revolver by his side and a steely resolve in his heart, Luke embarked on a perilous journey to confront The Reaper and his gang head-on. Along the way, he faced trials and tribulations beyond imagining, from fierce gunfights in the dusty streets to treacherous ambushes in the dead of night.

But with each passing day, Luke grew ever closer to his quarry, his determination unwavering in the face of adversity. And when the final showdown came, amidst the swirling dust and echoing gunfire, Luke stood tall against The Reaper and his minions, his courage shining like a beacon of hope in the darkest of times.

In the end, as the last of The Reaper's gang lay defeated and broken, Sundown breathed a sigh of relief, its people free from the grip of fear that had held them captive for so long. And though the scars of The Reaper's reign would never fully heal, they served as a reminder of the strength and resilience of those who called Sundown home.

48. Thundering Wheel

The land stretched endlessly and danger lurked around every bend in the rugged expanse of the West, where. This was true the town of Rockridge as it was for any town. It was a place where the sun beat down mercilessly and the wind whispered tales of the frontier's secrets.

But Rockridge was not without its share of troubles, for it was besieged by bandits and outlaws who preyed on the unsuspecting travelers who passed through its streets. And in times of peril, there was one man who could always be counted on to deliver justice—Ethan Hayes, the town's fearless stagecoach driver.

With his trusty team of horses and nerves of steel, Ethan raced across the unforgiving terrain, his stagecoach thundering down the dusty trails like a force of nature. Each day brought new challenges and dangers, from treacherous river crossings to sudden ambushes by bandits lying in wait.

But Ethan was undeterred, his determination unwavering as he pressed forward, his only thought to deliver his precious cargo safely to its destination. For nestled within the confines of his stagecoach lay a message of utmost importance—a missive that could mean the difference between life and death for those who awaited its arrival.

As the miles stretched on and the sun dipped low on the horizon, Ethan pushed his team harder, urging them onward with a fierce determination born of duty and honor. And when at last he reached his destination, weary but triumphant, he delivered his message with a sense of pride that only a true hero could know.

For in the heart of the West, where danger was ever-present and the odds were stacked against them, Ethan Hayes had proven himself to be more than just a stagecoach driver—he was a symbol of hope in a land where hope was often in short supply. And as he rode off into the sunset, his legacy lived on in the hearts of those he had sworn to protect.

49. A Widow's Resolve

The modest homestead of Sarah Morgan was a beacon of resilience. A widow left to fend for herself in a land where danger lurked around every corner, she had to make do as best she could.

Sarah had known her fair share of hardships since the passing of her husband, but none compared to the threat that now loomed on the horizon. A gang of outlaws, led by the ruthless Jake Thornton, had set their sights on her land, eager to claim it for their own.

But Sarah was not one to back down from a fight. With a rifle in hand and steely determination in her heart, she stood firm against the encroaching tide of lawlessness, ready to defend what was rightfully hers.

As the outlaws descended upon her homestead, their shouts and gunfire echoing through the canyon, Sarah stood her ground, her nerves steeling against the onslaught. With each shot fired and each blow struck, she fought with a ferocity born of desperation, unwilling to surrender to the forces of darkness that threatened to consume her.

But just as it seemed that all hope was lost, a lone figure emerged from the shadows, his gun blazing with righteous fury. It was the town sheriff, drawn by the sound of gunfire and the cry for help that had echoed across the valley.

Together, Sarah and the sheriff fought side by side, their bullets finding their mark and driving back the outlaws with a force that could not be denied. And when at last the dust settled and the smoke cleared, Sarah stood victorious, her homestead safe once more.

For in the heart of the West, where danger lurked at every turn, Sarah Morgan had proven herself to be more than just a widow—she was a symbol of strength and resilience in a land where only the strongest survived.

50. The Preacher's Redemption

In the sprawling expanse of the Western frontier, nestled amidst the jagged peaks of the Rockies, lay the bustling mining town of Sagebrush Falls. Here, where the promise of gold drew men from far and wide, corruption ran rampant like a river of poison through the heart of the community.

But amidst the chaos and lawlessness, there stood one man who refused to bow to the darkness that threatened to engulf his home. Reverend Samuel Carter, a man of unwavering faith and unyielding resolve, had dedicated his life to bringing the light of righteousness to the darkest corners of Sagebrush Falls.

For years, Reverend Carter had watched in sorrow as greed and vice tore at the fabric of his beloved town, turning neighbor against neighbor and sowing seeds of discord and despair. But he refused to stand idly by while evil triumphed over good.

With fire in his eyes and the word of God on his lips, Reverend Carter took to the streets, rallying the downtrodden and inspiring hope in the hearts of those who had long since lost faith. He preached of justice and mercy, of redemption and forgiveness, and his words stirred something deep within the souls of the people of Sagebrush Falls.

But the forces of darkness were not so easily vanquished, and as Reverend Carter delved deeper into the heart of the corruption that gripped his town, he found himself facing adversaries more powerful and more ruthless than he could have ever imagined.

Yet, armed with nothing more than his unwavering faith and the courage of his convictions, Reverend Carter stood firm against the tide of wickedness that threatened to overwhelm him. For he knew that so long as there was even a single spark of hope left in the hearts of the people of Sagebrush Falls, there was still a chance for redemption—for himself, for his town, and for the soul of the West.

51. Pioneers of the Southwest

There were two brothers whose names would become synonymous with the spirit of the frontier. Their names were Charles and William Bent, pioneers and traders who carved a path through the wilderness.

Born into a world of uncertainty and adventure, Charles and William grew up along the banks of the Missouri River, where the call of the wild beckoned them to explore the untamed lands beyond. From a young age, they learned the ways of the land, mastering the skills of hunting, trapping, and survival that would serve them well in the years to come.

But it was their vision and entrepreneurial spirit that truly set the Bent brothers apart. In the early 19th century, as America expanded westward, they saw an opportunity to establish a trading empire in the heart of the Southwest—a gateway to the riches of the fur trade and a key player in the burgeoning commerce of the frontier.

With a combination of shrewd business acumen and fearless determination, Charles and William built Bent's Fort—a sprawling trading post and fortress that became a beacon of civilization in the wilds of the prairie. From its walls, they traded with Native American tribes, trappers, traders, and pioneers alike, forging alliances and building a reputation as fair and honest businessmen.

But amidst the hustle and bustle of frontier life, there were challenges and dangers aplenty. From conflicts with rival traders to skirmishes with hostile tribes, the Bent brothers faced countless obstacles on their journey to success. Yet through it all, they remained steadfast in their resolve, their bond as brothers and their shared vision guiding them through even the darkest of times.

And as the years passed and the West continued to change, the legacy of Charles and William Bent lived on—a demonstration of the pioneering spirit of those who dared to dream big and chase their dreams across the vast and untamed wilderness of the American frontier.

52. The Sharpshooter's Journey

Amidst the rugged plains of the Wild West, where dust devils danced across the arid landscape and the sun beat down with unrelenting force, there lived a young woman named Clara. With a heart full of ambition and eyes that gleamed with determination, she longed for a life beyond the confines of her small frontier town.

When a traveling Wild West show rolled into town, promising fame and fortune to those brave enough to join its ranks, Clara saw her chance to break free from the monotony of her daily life. With her father's old rifle slung over her shoulder and a fire burning in her soul, she set out to prove herself as the greatest sharpshooter the West had ever seen.

Under the guidance of the show's seasoned performers, Clara honed her skills with relentless dedication, her aim becoming as true as the North Star guiding her way. With each passing day, she grew stronger and more confident, her shots ringing out like thunder across the open plains.

But as the show traveled from town to town, entertaining crowds with death-defying feats of marksmanship and daring stunts, Clara soon found herself embroiled in a web of rivalry and betrayal that threatened to tear the troupe apart. Jealous performers sought to undermine her authority, while envious suitors vied for her affections, each one determined to see her fall.

Yet, despite the obstacles that stood in her way, Clara refused to be deterred. With nerves of steel and a steady hand, she faced each challenge head-on, her determination unwavering in the face of adversity.

And in the end, it was Clara's unwavering spirit and unyielding perseverance that earned her a place among the legends of the Wild West, her name spoken with reverence wherever tales of daring and adventure were told.

53. The Gold Hunter's Dilemma

Deep in the heart of the Mojave Desert, where the shimmering heatwaves danced across the horizon and the cacti stood sentinel against the relentless sun, there dwelled a man known as Jackson "Jacks" Reynolds. A weather-beaten prospector with a glint of determination in his eyes, Jacks had spent years combing the arid wasteland in search of his fortune.

One sweltering afternoon, as Jacks toiled beneath the blistering sun, his pickaxe struck something solid buried beneath the scorching sand. With bated breath, he uncovered a vein of gold that gleamed like a beacon in the desert heat. A surge of exhilaration coursed through his veins as he realized he had stumbled upon the mother lode.

But as news of Jacks' discovery spread throughout the frontier town of Dusty Creek, it attracted the attention of a band of ruthless claim jumpers led by the notorious outlaw, Black-eyed Pete. Determined to wrest Jacks' claim from his grasp, Pete and his gang descended upon the desert with guns blazing and malice in their hearts.

Refusing to relinquish his hard-earned prize without a fight, Jacks stood his ground against the marauding bandits, his trusty revolver at the ready. With nerves of steel and a steady hand, he faced down his adversaries in a showdown worthy of the Wild West legends.

Amidst the chaos of the gunfight, Jacks wrestled with a moral dilemma. Should he risk his life to protect his claim, or should he abandon his dreams of riches in the face of overwhelming odds? As bullets whizzed past his head and dust clouded his vision, he knew that his decision would determine his fate in the unforgiving frontier.

Jacks emerged victorious from the fray, his claim secured and his resolve unshaken. And as he gazed upon the glittering gold at his feet, he knew that no matter the challenges that lay ahead, he would always be a true son of the West—a man driven by courage, perseverance, and the unyielding spirit of adventure.

54. Trails of Longing

Kit was a solitary figure as he there rode across vast expanse of the untamed prairie. A rugged cowboy with a heart heavy with memories and a soul haunted by lost love, Kit had spent years roaming the open range in search of his one true companion.

It was on a moonlit night, as he sat beside his crackling campfire beneath a canopy of twinkling stars, that Kit's thoughts drifted back to the woman who had stolen his heart so many years ago. Her name was Sarah, a fiery-haired beauty with eyes as blue as the summer sky and a smile that could light up even the darkest of nights.

But fate had torn them apart, sending Sarah away to a distant town on the far side of the frontier, leaving Kit to wander the lonely trails of the West in search of solace. With each passing day, his longing for her grew stronger, until he could bear it no longer.

Determined to reunite with his lost love, Kit saddled his faithful steed and set out on a journey across the rugged terrain of the frontier. Through blistering heat and biting cold, he rode tirelessly, his heart filled with hope and determination.

As he crossed rivers and scaled mountains, Kit encountered bandits and bounty hunters, outlaws and lawmen, each one a reminder of the dangers that lurked around every bend in the trail. But nothing could deter him from his quest, for he knew that his destiny lay in the arms of the woman he loved.

Finally, after countless miles of hard riding, Kit arrived at the outskirts of Sarah's town, his heart pounding with anticipation. With a prayer on his lips and love in his heart, he urged his horse forward, ready to face whatever challenges lay ahead in his quest to find his long-lost love and reclaim the happiness that had eluded him for so long.

55. Shadows of the Sierra

Marshal Lucas Cutter squinted against the blazing sun as he rode through the rugged terrain of the Sierra Nevada Mountains, his steely gaze fixed on the rocky peaks looming overhead. For weeks, rumors had circulated about a notorious outlaw gang that had been terrorizing the nearby towns, their hideout rumored to be nestled deep within the maze of canyons and valleys that stretched across the rugged landscape.

Determined to bring the outlaws to justice, Cutter had assembled a small posse of seasoned lawmen and set out on a perilous journey into the heart of the wilderness. As they forged their way through dense forests and treacherous ravines, the marshal's thoughts were consumed by the task that lay ahead, his jaw set in grim determination.

Finally, after days of relentless pursuit, Cutter and his men stumbled upon the outlaws' hidden camp, nestled in a remote clearing at the base of a towering cliff. With the element of surprise on their side, the lawmen launched a swift and decisive assault, their guns blazing as they rode into the camp with guns drawn.

But the outlaws were ready for them, and a fierce gun battle erupted as bullets flew and shouts echoed through the canyon. Cutter fought with the ferocity of a man possessed, his senses sharpened by adrenaline as he exchanged gunfire with the gang's leader, a ruthless outlaw known only as "Haymaker" McPherson.

In the end, it was Cutter's unwavering resolve and iron will that won the day, as he single-handedly brought down McPherson and his gang, bringing an end to their reign of terror once and for all. As he stood victorious amid the smoldering ruins of the outlaw camp, Cutter knew that the mountains would hold their secrets no longer, and that justice had finally been served in the shadows of the Sierra.

56. Trails of Betrayal

The wagon train trudged along the dusty trail, the creaking of wooden wheels and the clip-clop of horses' hooves the only sounds breaking the eerie silence of the wilderness. Among the travelers were families seeking a new start in the West, their hopes and dreams tied to the promise of a better life on the frontier.

But their journey took a dark turn when a band of outlaws descended upon them like vultures, their faces obscured by bandanas as they rode out of the shadows, guns blazing. The peaceful tranquility of the trail was shattered by the chaos of gunfire and screams as the outlaws unleashed their fury upon the unsuspecting travelers.

In the midst of the chaos, a handful of survivors banded together, their resolve hardened by the desperate struggle for survival. With bullets whizzing past their heads and their hearts pounding in their chests, they fought tooth and nail to fend off their attackers and reach safety.

Leading the charge was Jed Morgan, a grizzled old prospector with a quick trigger finger and a fierce determination to see his companions through to the end. With his trusty rifle in hand, he picked off the outlaws one by one, his steely gaze never wavering as he guided the survivors through the treacherous terrain.

But the outlaws were relentless, their numbers seemingly endless as they closed in on the beleaguered travelers. With each passing mile, the odds grew more dire, and the line between life and death blurred ever further.

Yet despite the overwhelming odds stacked against them, the survivors refused to give up hope, their spirits buoyed by the unwavering camaraderie and determination to see their journey through to the end. And as the sun dipped below the horizon and the dust settled on the trail, they emerged victorious, their spirits unbroken and their resolve stronger than ever before.

57. Shadows of Redemption

Some towns just seem forgotten by time, too remote to thrive, too needed to die. This was such a town. Its streets were empty, save for the occasional tumbleweed that drifted lazily in the breeze, and its buildings stood weathered and worn, a testament to the hardships of life on the frontier.

It was here that Jake Dawson, a gunslinger with a troubled past and a heavy heart, sought refuge from the demons that haunted him. With every step he took, the weight of his sins bore down upon him, a constant reminder of the lives he had taken and the pain he had caused.

But despite his best efforts to leave his past behind, the shadows of his past followed him wherever he went, lurking in the corners of his mind and haunting his every waking moment. Try as he might to drown out the memories with whiskey and solitude, they clawed at him relentlessly, refusing to be forgotten.

It wasn't until he stumbled upon the remote town nestled in the heart of the desert that Jake found a glimmer of hope amidst the darkness that consumed him. With its quiet streets and welcoming inhabitants, it offered him a chance at redemption, a chance to leave his past behind and start anew.

But redemption was not easily won, and Jake soon found himself embroiled in the town's struggles, forced to confront the ghosts of his past and the demons that threatened to consume him. With each passing day, he fought tooth and nail to atone for his sins, to make amends for the lives he had taken and the pain he had caused.

And though the road to redemption was long and fraught with danger, Jake pressed on, fueled by the hope that one day, he might find peace amidst the chaos of the frontier.

58. Frontier Standoff

Frontiers are dangerous places, dangerous for the settlers and for the native people. It seemed the wind whispered tales of both danger and opportunity, for here lay a small settlement on the edge of the frontier. Its inhabitants, a group of hardy settlers seeking a new beginning in the uncharted territories, had carved out a meager existence amidst the harsh landscape, building their homes and tilling the land with hopes of a better future.

But their dreams of prosperity were soon shattered when rumors spread of a tribe of hostile Indians lurking in the surrounding wilderness, their intentions unknown and their numbers formidable. Fear gripped the settlement like a vice as the settlers braced themselves for the inevitable confrontation, knowing that their very survival depended on their ability to defend their homes and families against the impending threat.

As tensions mounted and nerves frayed, the settlers prepared for the battle that loomed on the horizon, knowing that they faced a formidable adversary in the warriors who prowled the shadows of the surrounding forest. With rifles in hand and hearts heavy with determination, they stood ready to make a stand against the forces that sought to drive them from their land and destroy everything they had worked so hard to build.

But as the sun dipped below the horizon and darkness descended upon the frontier, the settlers found themselves facing a difficult decision. Would they stand their ground and fight for their homes and families, or would they abandon everything they had worked so hard to achieve and flee into the unknown?

With their future hanging in the balance, the settlers steeled themselves for the battle ahead, knowing that their fate would be decided by the choices they made in the crucible of the frontier.

59. The Witness

In the quiet town of Hollow Springs, nestled amidst the rolling plains of the western frontier, young Tommy Jenkins spent his days roaming the dusty streets, his wide eyes filled with wonder at the world around him. But one fateful afternoon, his innocent wanderings led him to a sight that would haunt him forever.

As the sun dipped low on the horizon, casting long shadows across the deserted streets, Tommy stumbled upon a scene that would change his life forever. Hidden behind a dilapidated barn, he watched in horror as a shadowy figure emerged from the darkness, a gun glinting in the fading light. With a sudden burst of violence, the figure unleashed a hail of bullets, cutting down an unsuspecting victim in cold blood.

Frozen in terror, Tommy watched in silence as the murderer disappeared into the night, leaving behind nothing but death and destruction in his wake. With trembling hands and a pounding heart, he knew that he had witnessed something that he could never forget.

As word spread of the brutal murder that had rocked the small town, Tommy found himself thrust into the spotlight, his young voice suddenly at the the center of a storm of controversy. With the eyes of the entire town upon him, he knew that he had a choice to make: to stay silent and live with the guilt of knowing the truth, or to stand up and speak out, no matter the consequences.

With courage beyond his years, Tommy took the stand in a crowded courtroom, his voice steady as he recounted the horrors he had witnessed on that fateful night. And as his words rang out into the silence, he knew that he had done the right thing, no matter the cost. For in that moment, he had become more than just a witness to a crime – he had become a beacon of hope in a town shrouded in darkness.

60. The Raid

In the quiet, dusty town of Sagebrush Junction, the sun hung low on the horizon, casting long shadows across the deserted streets. The locals had retired to their homes for the evening, leaving the town seemingly empty. Little did they know, trouble was brewing at the bank.

A group of outlaws, their faces concealed by bandanas, crept through the alleys, their footsteps muffled by the soft layer of sand. They were on a mission, one that promised riches beyond their wildest dreams.

The leader, a grizzled man known only as Slim, approached the bank with cautious determination. His companions fanned out, keeping watch for any signs of trouble. With a swift motion, Slim pried open the back door of the bank, revealing the dimly lit interior.

Inside, the bank's lone teller, a young man named Jake, sat counting the day's earnings. He looked up in shock as the outlaws burst in, their guns drawn and ready for action.

"Hands up!" Slim barked, his voice rough and commanding. "This is a robbery!"

Jake complied, his hands shaking as he raised them above his head. The outlaws wasted no time, emptying the bank's vault of its contents and stuffing the stolen money into canvas sacks.

As they made their escape, the sound of gunfire echoed through the streets, alerting the townsfolk to the crime in progress. By the time the sheriff and his deputies arrived, the outlaws were long gone, leaving nothing but chaos and confusion in their wake.

For the people of Sagebrush Junction, it was a rude awakening to the harsh realities of life on the frontier. But for Slim and his gang, it was just another successful heist in a long line of criminal exploits.

61. Redemption Calls

Deputy Charles Drum squinted against the relentless glare of the setting sun as he rode into the dusty town of Redemption. The weight of his badge felt heavier than ever, each clinking step of his horse a reminder of the past he thought he'd left behind.

In Redemption, whispers lingered like ghosts among the wooden storefronts. Whispers of a man who once wore the same badge as Charles, a man with a reputation stained in blood and regret. A man Charles knew all too well — himself, before he turned his back on the darkness that consumed him.

But the past is a relentless pursuer, and Charles's sins were not easily outrun. As the shadows grew longer, so did the memories of the lives he'd taken, the choices that haunted his dreams.

It wasn't long before Redemption's tranquility was shattered by the arrival of a notorious outlaw gang, led by a face from Charles's past. The deputy's heart clenched in dread as he recognized the cold eyes of his former partner, Luke Thornton, now a wanted man with a price on his head.

Charles knew what he had to do. With a grim determination, he squared his shoulders and faced the demons he'd long tried to outrun. The dusty streets erupted in gunfire as Charles and Luke met in a showdown, the echoes of their past echoing in every shot fired.

In the end, only one man walked away from the chaos of Redemption, but both were forever changed. For Charles Drum, the shadows of his past had finally been confronted, and in the smoke-filled air of Redemption, he found the redemption he'd been seeking all along.

62. Blood Oath

In the unforgiving expanse of the Wild West, justice was often found at the barrel of a gun. Lucas Kane rode alone. His brother's blood still stained the earth, an unyielding testament to the brutality of those who had taken him.

Lucas was no stranger to the ways of the gun; he was a gunslinger feared by many, respected by few. But now, his only purpose was vengeance. He had made a promise at his brother's graveside, a solemn oath to hunt down the men responsible and deliver justice with unflinching resolve.

Tracking his prey through rugged terrain and barren deserts, Lucas's steely determination never wavered. He rode with the fury of a storm, fueled by grief and righteous anger.

Finally, he found them holed up in a ramshackle hideout, their faces twisted with arrogance and malice. Without hesitation, Lucas confronted them, his gun drawn with deadly precision.

The ensuing showdown was a symphony of gunfire and dust, each shot a testament to the thirst for retribution burning within Lucas's soul. In the chaos that ensued, justice was served with ruthless efficiency. One by one, the men who had robbed Lucas of his brother fell to the cold steel of his revolver.

As the dust settled and silence descended upon the scene, Lucas stood alone amidst the carnage, his heart heavy with the weight of his actions. But amidst the bloodshed, he found a measure of solace, knowing that his brother's memory had been avenged.

With one final glance at the horizon, Lucas holstered his weapon and rode off into the sunset, a lone figure in a vast and unforgiving land. Though the scars of his past would never fade, he carried with him the knowledge that he had fulfilled his blood oath, and in doing so, had found a semblance of peace in a world consumed by violence.

63. Hearts on the Range

On the sprawling expanse of the Double Diamond Ranch, nestled beneath the endless stretch of the Texas sky, lived the spirited and headstrong Lily Morgan. Daughter of the esteemed rancher, John Morgan, Lily was as wild and untamed as the land she called home.

It was amidst the golden fields and whispering winds that Lily's heart was captured by the rugged charm of Jesse Thompson, a cowboy from the rival Thompson Ranch. Their love was forbidden, a flame born from the embers of feuding families and bitter rivalries.

Despite the simmering tensions between their kin, Lily and Jesse found solace in stolen moments beneath the starlit canopy of the night sky. Their love blossomed like wildflowers in the spring, defying the boundaries that sought to keep them apart.

But as whispers of their forbidden romance spread like wildfire through the town, tensions reached a boiling point. The divide between the Morgan and

Thompson families seemed insurmountable, threatening to tear apart the fragile bond between Lily and Jesse.

In the face of adversity, Lily and Jesse clung to each other with unwavering devotion, determined to prove that love could conquer even the deepest of divides. With each passing day, their resolve grew stronger, their love burning bright amidst the shadows of uncertainty.

And when the time came to choose between loyalty to their families and loyalty to their hearts, Lily and Jesse knew that they could only follow the path that led them to each other.

In a world where boundaries were defined by fences and traditions, Lily and Jesse dared to defy the odds, forging a love that would endure the test of time. For in each other's arms, they found a sanctuary amidst the chaos of the world—a love that was as boundless and untamed as the open range itself.

64. Guardian of the Trail

A lone gunslinger rode alongside a weary wagon train. His name was Ethan Cross, a man of few words and steely resolve, known throughout the land as the Guardian of the Trail.

As the wagon train creaked and groaned its way across the vast and unforgiving terrain, whispers of impending danger echoed among the settlers. Outlaws, drawn by the promise of riches and fueled by greed, lurked in the shadows, ready to strike at any moment.

But Ethan Cross was a sentinel of the frontier, a guardian sworn to protect those who journeyed under his watchful eye. With nerves of steel and a steady hand, he stood as a bulwark against the tide of lawlessness that threatened to engulf the trail.

Time and again, the outlaws descended upon the wagon train like vultures, their guns blazing and their hearts filled with malice. But each time, they were met with the unyielding fury of Ethan Cross, a force of nature determined to defend the innocent at any cost.

In the blistering heat of the desert sun and the biting cold of the mountain passes, Ethan fought with a ferocity born of righteousness. His bullets found their mark with unerring precision, his presence striking fear into the hearts of those who dared to challenge him.

As the days turned into weeks and the miles stretched ever onward, the wagon train pressed forward under the watchful gaze of their guardian. And though the journey was fraught with peril and uncertainty, they found solace in the knowledge that Ethan Cross rode by their side, a silent sentinel standing between them and the abyss.

In the end, it was not the outlaws who prevailed, but the indomitable spirit of those who refused to yield to fear. And as the wagon train reached its destination, weary but unbowed, they looked back upon the trail they had traveled and whispered words of gratitude to the man who had become their savior—the Guardian of the Trail, Ethan Cross.

65. Rush Against Time

In Sierra Nevada a lone prospector named Samuel Cole stumbled upon a vein of gold that glittered like the promise of a new dawn.

With hands calloused from years of toil and eyes alight with newfound hope, Samuel knew that he had unearthed a fortune that could change his life forever. But in the unforgiving world of prospecting, time was a merciless adversary, and Samuel's claim was in peril.

As he gazed upon the golden bounty that lay before him, Samuel's heart raced with a mix of excitement and dread. For he knew that every passing moment brought the threat of rival prospectors and unscrupulous opportunists who would stop at nothing to steal his claim.

With a steely resolve born of desperation, Samuel gathered his meager belongings and set off on a treacherous journey back to town. Every step was a battle against the clock, the weight of his discovery pressing down upon him like a burden too heavy to bear.

Through rocky canyons and raging rivers, Samuel pushed himself to the brink of exhaustion, his every breath a prayer to the gods of fortune. And as the sun dipped below the horizon and darkness descended upon the land, he knew that time was running out.

But just when it seemed that all hope was lost, Samuel emerged from the wilderness and stumbled into the welcoming glow of civilization. With trembling hands and a heart pounding with relief, he made his way to the office of the land commissioner, where he filed his claim with trembling hands.

As the ink dried on the parchment and the weight of his triumph settled upon him, Samuel Cole knew that he had defied the odds and emerged victorious. For in the crucible of the wilderness, he had proven that fortune favored the bold, and that even in the face of insurmountable odds, there was always a chance to strike gold.

66. Message of Fate

In the bustling telegraph office of a small frontier town, the rhythmic clacking of keys echoed through the dimly lit room as Harold Monroe, the seasoned telegraph operator, sat hunched over his machine. His weathered fingers danced across the keys with practiced precision, transmitting messages that connected the isolated town to the outside world.

But on this fateful evening, amidst the static crackle of the wires and the hum of machinery, Harold received a message that would change the course of history for the town and its inhabitants.

With bated breath, he decoded the urgent dispatch, his heart pounding in his chest as he read the words that scrolled across the ticker tape. It was news of a coming storm, a tempest of unparalleled fury that threatened to unleash its wrath upon the unsuspecting town.

With a sense of urgency that bordered on desperation, Harold sprang into action, his fingers flying across the keys as he relayed the warning to the townsfolk. Through the night, he worked tirelessly, transmitting messages of evacuation and preparedness, his voice a beacon of hope amidst the encroaching darkness.

As the storm loomed ever closer, the townspeople rallied together, heeding Harold's warning and bracing themselves for the inevitable onslaught. Through the howling winds and crashing thunder, they stood united, their spirits unbroken by the fury of nature.

And when the storm finally passed, leaving destruction in its wake, the town emerged battered but unbroken, its resilience a testament to the power of community in the face of adversity.

In the aftermath of the chaos, Harold Monroe returned to his telegraph office, his fingers poised over the keys once more. Though the storm had passed, his work was far from over. For in the quiet moments between messages, he knew that the next dispatch could bring news of hope or despair, shaping the fate of the town and its people with every word transmitted across the wires.

67. Trails of the Market

As the first light of dawn painted the sky with hues of orange and gold, Jeb Parker, a seasoned cowboy, saddled his horse and prepared to embark on the long journey from the ranch to the bustling market town. With a whistle on his lips and the steady rhythm of hooves beneath him, Jeb set out on the trail, his faithful cattle trailing behind like a river of living, breathing wealth.

Through rugged canyons and rolling hills, Jeb guided his herd with a practiced hand, his eyes scanning the horizon for signs of trouble. Jeb was no stranger to adversity. With nerves of steel and a heart as vast as the open range, he led his cattle with his determination unwavering in the face of hardship.

As the days turned into weeks and the miles stretched ever onward, Jeb and his herd pressed forward with unwavering resolve. Each step brought them closer to their destination, to the promise of profit and prosperity that awaited them in the market town.

And when they finally arrived, dusty and weary but unbowed, Jeb felt a swell of pride in his chest as he watched his cattle being unloaded and herded into the pens. For in that moment, he knew that his hard work had paid off, that he had brought his livestock safely to market and ensured a profitable return for the ranch.

As the sun dipped below the horizon and the market bustled with activity, Jeb leaned against the corral fence and watched with a sense of satisfaction. For though the journey had been long and arduous, the rewards were worth every hardship endured along the way.

And as he rode back to the ranch beneath the starlit sky, Jeb Parker knew that he was more than just a cowboy—he was a steward of the land, a guardian of the herd, and a master of the trails that stretched across the untamed frontier.

68. The Last Ride of George Willis

In the unforgiving expanse of the Wild West, where the echoes of gunfire sometimes rang through the canyons, George Willis rode with a heart heavy with grief and a soul ablaze with vengeance.

It had been months since the brutal massacre that had torn his family apart, leaving George alone in a world consumed by violence and lawlessness. But he was no stranger to the ways of the gun, no stranger to the harsh realities of life on the frontier.

With every mile he rode, George's resolve grew stronger, fueled by the memory of his loved ones and the burning desire for justice. He tracked the outlaws who had robbed him of everything he held dear with unwavering determination, his eyes set on the horizon like a hunter stalking his prey.

Through dust-choked canyons and sun-baked plains, George pursued his quarry, his heart a furnace of rage and sorrow. And when he finally found them holed up in a remote outlaw camp, he knew that the time for vengeance had come.

The ensuing showdown was a whirlwind of violence and chaos, bullets tearing through the air like angry hornets as George faced off against the men who had taken everything from him. But in the end, there was only one man left standing amidst the carnage—the lone figure of George Willis, bathed in the light of the setting sun.

As he surveyed the aftermath of the battle, George felt a sense of emptiness wash over him, the weight of his actions heavy on his shoulders. For though he had avenged his family's death, he knew that no amount of bloodshed could ever bring them back.

With a heavy heart and a weary soul, George Willis mounted his horse and rode off into the fading light, leaving behind the wreckage of his past and the ghosts that haunted his dreams. And as he disappeared into the vastness of the wilderness, he knew that his journey was far from over, that the road ahead would be long and fraught with peril.

But wherever the trail may lead him, George Willis would ride on, a solitary figure in a world consumed by darkness, forever seeking redemption amidst the shadows of the Wild West.

69. Lessons of the Heart

As the sun dipped low over the horizon, casting hues of gold and crimson across the vast expanse of the Western frontier, Emily Caldwell stepped off the stagecoach in the bustling town of Willow Creek. With determination in her heart and a passion for education, she had journeyed from the East to pursue her dream of teaching in the untamed wilderness of the West.

Settling into her role as the new schoolteacher, Emily quickly endeared herself to the townsfolk with her warmth and dedication. Yet amidst the flurry of lessons and laughter, it was the enigmatic William Buxton who caught her eye—a rugged cowboy with a heart as vast as the prairie sky.

Their first encounter was a chance meeting at the town's general store, where William's easy smile and genuine kindness left Emily breathless. From that moment on, their paths seemed destined to intertwine, like two rivers converging in the vastness of the wilderness.

As they spent more time together, Emily and William discovered a shared love for the land and a deep connection that defied explanation. Amidst moonlit walks beneath the towering cottonwoods and stolen glances, their bond blossomed like wildflowers in the spring.

Young love led to marriage as their love grew strong every day.

As they stood beneath the endless canopy of stars, Emily and William knew that their love was a force as timeless and enduring as the land itself. And as they looked toward the horizon, where the sun rose anew with each passing day, they knew that their journey together was only just beginning.

70. Tales from the Mississippi

Word had spread like wildfire through the streets of Stanley Falls - Mark Twain was coming to town.

As the sun dipped below the horizon, casting long shadows over the sleepy town, the stage was set for an evening of laughter and storytelling. In the dimly lit hall of the Stanly Falls Community Hall, rows of wooden chairs awaited their eager occupants, while the stage stood adorned with a simple podium and a single chair.

And then, amidst a swell of applause and cheers, he appeared—Mark Twain, the legendary humorist and raconteur, his white suit gleaming in the soft glow of lamplight. With a twinkle in his eye and a wry smile playing at the corners of his lips, he took his place behind the podium, his presence commanding the attention of all who had gathered to hear him speak.

For hours, Mark regaled the audience with tales of his travels along the mighty Mississippi, spinning yarns of steamboat races and riverboat gamblers, of larger-than-life characters and narrow escapes. With each word he spoke, he transported his listeners to a bygone era, where the sound of paddlewheels echoed through the night and the promise of adventure lurked around every bend in the river.

But amidst the laughter and applause, there was an undercurrent of something deeper—a message woven into the fabric of Mark's stories, a reflection on the human condition and the timeless truths that bind us all together.

And as the evening drew to a close and the audience reluctantly rose from their seats, they carried with them not just memories of laughter and joy, but a newfound appreciation for the power of storytelling to bridge the gap between past and present, between dreams and reality.

For in the words of Mark Twain, they had found not just entertainment, but a glimpse into the heart and soul of a nation—a nation bound together by the mighty Mississippi and the stories that flowed from its shores.

71. Geronimo's Legacy

In the rugged terrain of the American Southwest, there lived a man whose name struck fear into the hearts of settlers and soldiers alike. His name was Geronimo.

Born into the Bedonkohe band of the Apache tribe, Geronimo was raised on the principles of courage, honor, and resilience. From a young age, he learned the ways of the warrior, honing his skills in battle and mastering the art of survival in the unforgiving wilderness.

But as the tide of history shifted and the lands of his ancestors were encroached upon by settlers and soldiers, Geronimo found himself thrust into a conflict that would define his legacy for generations to come.

With unmatched ferocity and unyielding determination, Geronimo led his people in a relentless campaign of resistance against the forces of colonization. From the rocky cliffs of the Sierra Madre to the scorched valleys of the Sonoran Desert, he waged a guerrilla war against overwhelming odds, striking fear into the hearts of his enemies with lightning raids and sudden ambushes.

But Geronimo was more than just a warrior—he was a leader, a visionary, a symbol of hope for his people in their darkest hour. Despite the countless betrayals and broken promises he endured, he never wavered in his commitment to defending his homeland and preserving the Apache way of life.

And though the battles he fought may have been lost, Geronimo's spirit remained unbroken. Even in defeat, he refused to surrender to despair, continuing to resist with a tenacity that defied all logic and reason.

In the end, Geronimo's legacy was not one of conquest or defeat, but of resilience and perseverance in the face of overwhelming adversity. His name would be remembered not as a symbol of fear, but as a beacon of hope for future generations—a reminder that even in the darkest of times, the spirit of freedom and independence could never be extinguished.

72. Lawman's Redemption

In the heart of the wild frontier lay the town of Bitter Creek, where the law was as scarce as water in a drought. Sheriff Sam Walker was the exception, a lone beacon of justice in a sea of corruption.

For years, Bitter Creek had been ruled by the iron fist of the ruthless land baron, Silas McCallister. Under his tyrannical reign, the townsfolk lived in fear, and justice was nothing but a forgotten dream.

But Sheriff Walker refused to turn a blind eye to the injustices that plagued his town. With grit and determination, he fought tooth and nail to uphold the law, even in the face of overwhelming odds.

Day by day, Sheriff Walker chipped away at McCallister's stranglehold on Bitter Creek, arresting his cronies and bringing them to justice one by one. But the road to redemption was paved with blood and sacrifice, and Sheriff Walker knew that he would have to pay the price for his defiance.

As tensions reached a boiling point, Sheriff Walker found himself standing alone against McCallister and his hired guns. In a showdown that would decide the fate of Bitter Creek, he stared down the barrel of a dozen rifles, his hand poised over his trusty Colt.

With nerves of steel, Sheriff Walker faced his adversaries head-on, refusing to back down in the face of overwhelming odds. In a thunderous exchange of gunfire, justice was served, and Bitter Creek was finally free from the grip of tyranny.

As the dust settled and the echoes of gunfire faded into the wind, Sheriff Walker stood tall, a symbol of hope and resilience in a town that had lost its way. And though the scars of battle would never fade, Bitter Creek would rise from the ashes, stronger and more united than ever before.

73. The Legacy of Sitting Bull

In the vast expanse of the Great Plains, where the wind whispered ancient secrets and the earth echoed with the hoofbeats of buffalo, there lived a man whose name was spoken with reverence and respect. His name was Sitting Bull, a Sioux chief whose wisdom and courage had made him a legend among his people.

From a young age, Sitting Bull had been destined for greatness. Born into the Hunkpapa band of the Lakota Sioux, he quickly distinguished himself as a leader and a visionary, his keen insight and unwavering resolve guiding his people through times of hardship and strife.

But it was his defiance in the face of adversity that truly set Sitting Bull apart. When the encroachment of white settlers threatened to engulf his people's way of life, he refused to back down, rallying his warriors to defend their ancestral lands with fierce determination.

Despite facing overwhelming odds, Sitting Bull led his people to victory time and again, his strategic brilliance and unwavering courage earning him a place in history as one of the greatest Native American leaders of all time.

But Sitting Bull's legacy extended far beyond the battlefield. He was a man of peace as well as war, a seeker of truth and justice in a world torn apart by conflict and division. Through his words and actions, he sought to bridge the gap between cultures, to find common ground amidst the turmoil of the times.

And though his life was cut short by violence, his spirit lived on in the hearts of his people, a beacon of hope and inspiration for generations to come. For Sitting Bull was more than just a chief—he was a symbol of resilience and strength, a testament to the enduring spirit of the Lakota Sioux and the indomitable human will to persevere in the face of adversity.

74. Custer's Last Stand

In the sprawling expanse of the Great Plains there lived a man whose name would live forever. His name was General George Armstrong Custer, a cavalry officer whose daring exploits and reckless ambition had made him both a hero and a sometimes controversial figure.

From the battlefields of the Civil War to the untamed wilderness of the West, Custer had carved a reputation for himself as a fearless leader, his flamboyant style and unwavering confidence earning him the admiration of his men and the attention of the nation.

But it was his final campaign that would cement his place in history. In the summer of 1876, Custer led the 7th Cavalry on an expedition into the heart of Sioux territory, determined to crush the resistance of the Native American tribes and secure victory for the United States.

But what awaited him at the Little Bighorn River was a force far greater than he could have imagined. Thousands of Sioux and Cheyenne warriors, led by the legendary Sitting Bull and Crazy Horse, lay in wait, their numbers outnumbering Custer's troops by a significant margin.

Undeterred by the odds stacked against him, Custer ordered a reckless charge against the Native American encampment, confident in his ability to achieve a swift and decisive victory. But what followed was a massacre of unimaginable proportions, as Custer and his men were overwhelmed by the sheer force of the enemy's onslaught.

In the end, Custer's last stand would go down in history as one of the most infamous military defeats in American history. But amidst the tragedy and loss, his legacy would endure—a testament to the courage and determination of a man who dared to defy the odds, even in the face of certain death.

75. Annie's Aim

In the Wild West, there was a sharpshooter whose name was whispered with awe and admiration. Her name was Annie Oakley, and she was a legend in her own right.

From the moment she picked up her first rifle, Annie's aim was true, her eyes keen and her hands steady as she honed her skills on the rolling plains of Ohio. With each shot fired, she proved herself to be a force to be reckoned with—a woman who could outshoot even the most seasoned of marksmen.

But it was her time with Buffalo Bill's Wild West Show that would truly catapult Annie to fame and fortune. As a star attraction, she dazzled audiences with her precision and prowess, her feats of marksmanship leaving crowds breathless and begging for more.

Yet amidst the glare of the spotlight, Annie remained humble and down-to-earth, her heart always true to her roots. For beneath the glitz and glamour of show business, she was still the same girl from the Ohio countryside, with a love for the land and a spirit as wild as the open prairie.

But Annie's greatest legacy was not her skill with a rifle, but her unwavering courage and determination in the face of adversity. Despite facing countless challenges and setbacks throughout her life, she never lost sight of her dreams, never gave up on her quest to prove that a woman could do anything a man could do—and do it even better.

And though she may have passed into legend, Annie Oakley's spirit lives on in the hearts of all who dare to dream, a reminder that with perseverance and determination, anything is possible. For Annie's aim was not just true—it was unstoppable.

76. Buffalo Bill's Royal Performance

In the bustling streets of London, where the fog hung heavy and the sound of carriage wheels echoed through the cobblestone alleys, excitement rippled through the air like electricity. For the great showman, Buffalo Bill Cody, was coming to town, and with him, he brought the untamed spirit of the American West.

As news of his arrival spread like wildfire through the city, anticipation mounted among the citizens of London. Never before had they witnessed the spectacle of the Wild West—the thundering hooves of buffalo, the crack of bullwhips, the daring feats of marksmanship that seemed to defy all logic and reason.

But it was not just the common folk who were eager to see Buffalo Bill's show. Even Queen Victoria herself had expressed a keen interest in experiencing the wonders of the American frontier firsthand—a request that Cody was all too happy to oblige.

And so, on a cool autumn evening, under the watchful gaze of Buckingham Palace, Buffalo Bill's Wild West Show came to life before a royal audience unlike any other. The Queen herself, dressed in her finest attire, sat enthralled as cowboys and Indians rode across the makeshift arena, their lassos spinning and rifles firing in a dazzling display of skill and precision.

For hours, the spectacle continued—a whirlwind of excitement and wonder that transported the audience to a world far removed from the hustle and bustle of city life. From daring bronco riders to graceful trick ropers, each act seemed to outshine the last, leaving the spectators breathless with awe and admiration.

But perhaps the most memorable moment of the evening came when Buffalo Bill himself took to the stage, his presence commanding the attention of all who beheld him. With a twinkle in his eye and a smile on his lips, he regaled the audience with tales of his adventures on the American frontier, his larger-than-life persona filling the arena with a sense of excitement and wonder.

As the final curtain fell and the crowd erupted into applause, Queen Victoria rose from her seat, a smile playing at the corners of her lips. For in Buffalo Bill's Wild West Show, she had witnessed not just a spectacle, but a celebration of the human spirit—a testament to the indomitable courage and resilience of the American pioneers who had carved a legacy out of the untamed wilderness. And as she left the arena that night, her heart filled with memories of the sights and sounds of the Wild West, she knew that she had experienced something truly extraordinary—a once-in-a-lifetime adventure that would stay with her forever.

77. Billy's Last Ride

In the streets of Lincoln County, New Mexico, there lived a young man whose name struck fear into the hearts of lawmen and outlaws alike. His name was Billy the Kid, a notorious gunslinger whose legend would echo through history for generations to come.

From a young age, Billy had known the harsh realities of life on the frontier. Born into poverty and raised in the crucible of violence, he had learned to fend for himself from an early age, his quick wit and even quicker trigger finger earning him a reputation as a force to be reckoned with.

But it was not until the Lincoln County War that Billy's legend truly began to take shape. Faced with corruption and injustice on all sides, he took up arms alongside a band of fellow outlaws, determined to fight for what he believed was right, no matter the cost.

Yet amidst the chaos and bloodshed, there was a glimmer of humanity in Billy's heart—a sense of loyalty and camaraderie that belied his reputation as a cold-blooded killer. For amidst the violence and lawlessness of the frontier, he had found a family among the outlaws who rode by his side, a bond forged in the crucible of adversity.

But as the days turned into weeks and the law closed in around them, Billy knew that their days were numbered. With a heavy heart and a sense of resignation, he prepared for what would be his final ride—a desperate attempt to escape the long arm of the law and find freedom on the open range.

And so, as the sun dipped below the horizon and the stars began to twinkle in the night sky, Billy the Kid rode out of Lincoln County for the last time, his heart heavy with the weight of his deeds and the knowledge that his days were numbered.

But even as he rode into the darkness, Billy's legend lived on—a testament to the indomitable spirit of the American West and the men and women who dared to defy the odds in pursuit of a better life.

78. Wild Bill's Gamble

In the heart of the bustling frontier town of Deadwood, the saloons buzzed with the raucous laughter of miners and outlaws. Here there lived a man whose name struck fear into the hearts of those who crossed him. His name was Wild Bill Hickok, a legendary gunslinger whose reputation as a marksman was matched only by his love for gambling.

With a keen eye and nerves of steel, Wild Bill ruled the poker tables of Deadwood with a combination of skill and bravado that made him a force to be reckoned with. But it was not just his prowess with a gun that set him apart—it was his uncanny ability to read his opponents, to anticipate their every move before they even knew what hit them.

Yet amidst the chaos and excitement of the gambling halls, there was a darkness in Wild Bill's soul—a sense of emptiness that no amount of winnings could ever fill. For beneath the swagger and bravado lay a man haunted by his past, a man whose life had been touched by tragedy and loss.

But it was one fateful night in Deadwood that would change everything for Wild Bill. As he sat at the poker table, the cards falling in his favor with uncanny precision, he found himself face to face with a stranger whose eyes burned with a fire that matched his own.

With each hand dealt and each wager placed, the tension in the room grew thicker, until finally, there was only one hand left to play—a hand that would determine the fate of both men.

As the cards were revealed and the stakes were laid bare, Wild Bill knew that he was gambling not just with his money, but with his very life. For the stranger across the table was none other than Jack McCall, a desperate man with nothing left to lose.

And as the final card fell and the smoke cleared, it was Wild Bill who emerged victorious, his hand a winning combination that sealed his fate as one of the greatest gamblers the West had ever known.

But even in victory, there was a price to be paid—a price that Wild Bill would ultimately pay with his life.

For in the lawless town of Deadwood, where justice was often meted out at the end of a gun barrel, the line between life and death was as thin as a playing card, and sometimes, even the best hand wasn't enough to beat the odds.

79. The Outlaw's Legacy

His name was Jesse James, a notorious outlaw from Missouri whose name struck fear into the hearts of those who crossed his path.

From a young age, Jesse had been drawn to a life of crime, his rebellious spirit and quick temper leading him down a path of lawlessness and violence. Alongside his brother Frank and a band of fellow outlaws, he terrorized the countryside, robbing banks and stagecoaches with a daring and audacity that left lawmen scratching their heads in frustration.

But amidst the chaos and bloodshed, there was a complexity to Jesse's character—a sense of loyalty and honor that belied his reputation as a cold-blooded killer. For beneath the outlaw's exterior lay a man driven by a sense of justice, a man who saw himself as a champion of the downtrodden and oppressed.

Yet even as Jesse's exploits made him a folk hero among the common folk, they also made him a target for those who sought to bring him to justice. And so it was that on a fateful day in 1882, Jesse James met his end at the hands of a fellow outlaw—a betrayal that would seal his fate and cement his place in history as one of the most infamous outlaws of the American West.

But even in death, Jesse James's legacy lived on—a testament to the enduring allure of the outlaw and the untamed spirit of the frontier. For though he may have been a criminal in the eyes of the law, to those who revered him, Jesse James would forever be remembered as a symbol of freedom and rebellion in a land where the rules were made to be broken.

80. Remember the Alamo

In the heart of Texas, where the lone star shone bright in the vast expanse of the night sky, there stood a fortress whose name would forever be etched in the annals of history. Its name was the Alamo, a symbol of courage and sacrifice that would inspire generations to come.

In the early hours of March 6, 1836, the walls of the Alamo echoed with the sound of gunfire and the cries of battle as a small band of Texan defenders fought valiantly against overwhelming odds. Surrounded on all sides by the forces of General Santa Anna, they knew that their chances of survival were slim, yet still they refused to surrender.

For thirteen days and thirteen nights, the defenders of the Alamo held fast against wave after wave of Mexican soldiers, their determination unyielding in the face of certain death. Led by men like William B. Travis, Davy Crockett, and Jim Bowie, they stood as a beacon of hope in a land torn apart by revolution and war.

But in the end, the defenders of the Alamo could hold out no longer. Overwhelmed by sheer numbers and facing insurmountable odds, they fought to the last man, their sacrifice forever immortalized in the annals of Texas history.

Yet though they may have fallen, the spirit of the Alamo lived on—a rallying cry for those who sought freedom and independence from tyranny. For in their defiance and courage, the defenders of the Alamo had inspired a nation to rise up and fight for what they believed in, no matter the cost.

And so, as the lone star continued to shine over the land of Texas, the memory of the Alamo burned bright in the hearts of all who cherished freedom and democracy. For though the fortress may have fallen, its legacy would endure—a testament to the power of the human spirit and the enduring quest for liberty and justice for all.

81. The Cattle Baron's Guardian

The land stretched out like an endless sea of grass and the sun beat down mercilessly upon the earth, such was the frontier. There stood the sprawling ranch of the formidable cattle baron, Elijah Monk. His herds roamed freely across the open range, their lowing cries echoing through the valleys and canyons.

But with great wealth came great danger, and Elijah knew that his empire was under constant threat from rival ranchers, rustlers, and outlaws seeking to claim his riches for themselves. Determined to protect his interests at any cost, he turned to the only man he trusted to keep his cattle safe: the legendary gunslinger known only as "Iron" Billy Eastern.

Iron Billy was a man of few words and even fewer scruples, his reputation as deadly as the six-shooter that hung low on his hip. For a hefty sum of gold, he pledged his loyalty to Elijah Monk, vowing to defend his land and his livelihood with his very life if need be.

As the days turned into weeks and the weeks into months, Iron Billy rode tirelessly across the vast expanse of the Monk Ranch, his keen eyes ever watchful for signs of trouble on the horizon. He faced down rustlers and bandits with a cold and steely resolve, his lightning-fast draw striking fear into the hearts of those who dared to challenge him.

But as Iron Billy patrolled the borders of the Monk Ranch, he found himself drawn into a web of intrigue and treachery that threatened to consume him whole. Rival ranchers sought to undermine Elijah's authority, while whispers of rebellion spread like wildfire through the ranks of his own hired hands.

Yet, despite the dangers that lurked around every corner, Iron Billy remained steadfast in his duty to protect the cattle baron and his interests. For he knew that as long as he drew breath, the Monk Ranch would remain a fortress against the chaos of the wild frontier.

82. The Revolver's Revolution

Samuel Colt was the mastermind behind one of the most revolutionary inventions of his time—the Colt revolver.

From a young age, Samuel Colt showed a knack for tinkering and invention. Inspired by the workings of a ship's wheel, he devised a mechanism that would allow a firearm to fire multiple shots without the need for reloading—a concept that would change the course of history.

With determination and ingenuity, Colt set about refining his invention, perfecting the design and overcoming countless obstacles along the way. And in 1836, he unveiled his masterpiece to the world—the Colt Paterson revolver, a weapon that would revolutionize the way wars were fought and won.

From the battlefields of the American Civil War to the lawless streets of the Wild West, the Colt revolver became a symbol of power and authority, its sleek design and deadly accuracy making it the weapon of choice for soldiers, lawmen, and outlaws alike.

But Samuel Colt's legacy extended far beyond the realm of firearms. With his innovative manufacturing techniques and visionary approach to business, he laid the groundwork for modern industrial production, paving the way for a new era of technological advancement and economic prosperity.

And though he may have passed into history, Samuel Colt's influence can still be felt today—in the countless lives saved by his firearms, in the industries he helped to shape, and in the spirit of innovation and entrepreneurship that he embodied.

For Samuel Colt was more than just an inventor—he was a pioneer, a visionary, and a true trailblazer in every sense of the word. And though his name may have faded from memory, his legacy will endure as long as there are those who dream of progress.

83. Davy Crockett

From the untamed wilderness of Tennessee there came a man whose name would echo through the annals of history like a thunderclap. His name was Davy Crockett, a frontiersman, soldier, and folk hero whose legend would become inseparable from the spirit of the American frontier.

From humble beginnings in a log cabin deep in the backwoods, Davy Crockett forged a path through the wilderness with his rifle at his side and a twinkle in his eye. With a larger-than-life personality and a gift for storytelling, he quickly became a legend among his peers—a man whose exploits were the stuff of legend.

But it was on the battlefield where Davy Crockett would truly make his mark. As a soldier in the Tennessee militia and later in the Texas Revolution, he fought with a ferocity and courage that inspired all who fought alongside him. From the Siege of the Alamo to the Battle of San Jacinto, he led by example, rallying his comrades with his fearless spirit and unwavering resolve.

Yet amidst the chaos and bloodshed of war, there was a warmth and humanity to Davy Crockett that endeared him to all who knew him. Whether sharing a meal with his fellow soldiers or regaling them with tales of his adventures, he remained true to himself— a simple frontiersman with a heart as big as the wilderness he called home.

And though his life was cut short in the crucible of battle, Davy Crockett's legacy lived on—a testament to the indomitable spirit of the American frontier and the men and women who dared to tame it. For as long as there are those who cherish the spirit of adventure and the pursuit of freedom, the legend of Davy Crockett will endure, a beacon of hope and inspiration for generations to come.

84. The Lone Star Guardians

In the vast expanse of the Texas frontier there arose a band of men whose courage and resolve would come to embody the spirit of justice in the Wild West. They were the Texas Rangers, a legendary force of lawmen tasked with taming the untamed wilderness and bringing order to the lawless land.

Formed in the early days of the Republic of Texas, the Texas Rangers were a rugged and resourceful bunch, drawn from all walks of life and united by a common purpose—to protect the innocent and uphold the law, no matter the cost.

From their humble beginnings as a ragtag militia, the Texas Rangers quickly gained a reputation as some of the most feared and respected lawmen in the West. With their iconic silver stars glinting in the sunlight and their trusty six-shooters always at the ready, they rode out into the untamed wilderness, ready to face down bandits, outlaws, and hostile Native American tribes alike.

But it was not just their skill with a gun that set the Texas Rangers apart—it was their unwavering dedication to justice and their willingness to do whatever it took to see that justice served. Whether tracking down fugitives through the swamps of East Texas or standing firm against overwhelming odds in a shootout on the open range, the Texas Rangers never backed down from a challenge.

And though the days of the Wild West may be long gone, the legend of the Texas Rangers lives on—a tribute to the enduring spirit of the Lone Star State and the brave men who risked their lives to keep its citizens safe. For as long as there are those who dare to defy the law, there will always be the Texas Rangers, guardians of justice in the land of the lone star.

85. Savior of Crystal Rock

From the harrowing trails of the Civil War to the quiet streets of Crystal Rock, Captain Sam Lawson found himself at another frontier. His worn boots echoed as he strode down the wooden sidewalks, eyeing the rowdy saloons and wary locals.

Lawson's reputation preceded him, tales of his iron will and steadfastness spreading like wildfire. Crystal Rock, once a haven for outlaws, now trembled at the mere mention of his name.

The townsfolk watched with bated breath as Lawson imposed order with his weathered Colt at his side. He dispensed justice with a steady hand, earning respect even from those he jailed.

But beneath his steely exterior lay a man haunted by ghosts of the past. Memories of battlefields and fallen comrades weighed heavy on his soul. Yet, it was here in Crystal Rock that he found purpose once more.

One evening, a gang of desperados rode into town, their guns blazing and intent on wreaking havoc. Lawson stood firm, his eyes ablaze with determination as he faced down the outlaws.

In a showdown that echoed through the streets, Lawson emerged victorious, his reputation as a lawman cemented in the annals of Crystal Rock's history. The townsfolk hailed him as their savior, and for the first time in years, Lawson allowed himself a moment of solace.

As the sun dipped below the horizon, casting long shadows across the dusty plains, Captain Sam Lawson stood tall, a beacon of hope in the wild west.

86. The Denim Pioneer

In the bustling streets of San Francisco during the Gold Rush of the mid-19th century there lived a man whose name would become synonymous with durability, quality, and American ingenuity. His name was Levi Strauss, and he was the visionary behind one of the most iconic symbols of American culture—the blue jeans.

Born in Bavaria in 1829, Levi Strauss immigrated to the United States in search of opportunity and adventure. Settling in San Francisco, he established a successful dry goods business, supplying miners with everything they needed for their quest for gold.

But it was a chance encounter with a tailor from Nevada that would change the course of Levi Strauss's life forever. Hearing of the miners' need for durable work pants, Strauss began experimenting with different fabrics, eventually settling on a sturdy twilled cotton fabric known as denim.

In 1873, Levi Strauss and his partner, Jacob Davis, patented the design for the first-ever blue jeans, featuring riveted pockets and a reinforced waistband for extra strength. Almost overnight, the iconic pants became a hit among miners, cowboys, and laborers across the West, prized for their durability and rugged good looks.

But it was not just the practicality of Levi's jeans that made them a success—it was the sense of rugged individualism and freedom that they represented. From the cowboys of the Wild West to the rebels of the counterculture movement, Levi's jeans became a symbol of American identity and the spirit of adventure.

And though Levi Strauss himself may have passed into history, his legacy lives on in every pair of jeans bearing his name.

87. The Notorious James Gang

In the lawless expanse of the American Midwest during the late 19th century there roamed a band of outlaws whose name struck fear into the hearts of all who heard it. They were the James Gang, a notorious group of desperados led by the infamous Jesse James.

Born from the ashes of the Civil War, the James Gang was a force to be reckoned with—a ruthless band of bandits who plundered banks, stagecoaches, and trains with impunity, leaving a trail of destruction in their wake. With Jesse James at the helm, they struck fear into the hearts of law-abiding citizens and lawmen alike, their daring exploits making them the stuff of legend.

But beneath the veneer of outlawry lay a complex web of loyalties and betrayals. For while the James Gang may have been bound by blood and camaraderie, they were also driven by greed and ambition, with tensions simmering just beneath the surface.

As the law closed in around them and their notoriety grew, the James Gang became increasingly desperate, their robberies growing more audacious and their methods more violent. But even as they evaded capture time and time again, the end was drawing near.

In 1882, tragedy struck the James Gang when Jesse James was gunned down in his own home by a member of his own gang, seeking the reward money offered for his capture. With their leader dead and their ranks decimated, the remaining members of the James Gang scattered to the winds, their reign of terror coming to an abrupt and bloody end.

88. The Outlaw's Gambit

Dave Rudabaugh was an outlaw whose daring exploits would become the stuff of legend.

Born into poverty in Illinois, Dave Rudabaugh learned early on that the only law of the land was the law of survival. With a quick wit and a faster draw, he carved out a name for himself as a skilled gunman and a ruthless bandit, preying on travelers, stagecoaches, and trains with equal abandon.

But it was not just his skill with a gun that set Dave Rudabaugh apart—it was his audacity and cunning. With a keen eye for opportunity and a taste for danger, he orchestrated daring heists and brazen robberies that left lawmen scratching their heads in frustration.

Yet for all his bravado, Dave Rudabaugh was a man haunted by his own demons. With a price on his head and the law hot on his trail, he knew that his days were numbered. And so, in a desperate bid to escape the long arm of justice, he made a fateful decision—to join the infamous Lincoln County Regulators, a band of outlaws led by the notorious Billy the Kid.

But even amidst the chaos and violence of the Regulators, Dave Rudabaugh found himself drawn to a different path. As the law closed in around them and tensions within the gang reached a boiling point, he began to question his loyalty to Billy the Kid and the outlaw life.

And so, when the opportunity presented itself, Dave Rudabaugh made his move—a daring escape that would see him ride off into the sunset, leaving behind a trail of chaos and uncertainty in his wake. He was a symbol of defiance and rebellion in a land where the line between right and wrong was often blurred beyond recognition.

89. The Lawman's Legacy

Wyatt Earp was a legendary lawman whose courage and determination would make him a symbol of hope in a land where chaos reigned supreme.

From a young age, Wyatt Earp was drawn to the call of adventure and the thrill of the frontier. With a strong sense of justice and a steely resolve, he set out to make a name for himself as a peacekeeper and defender of the innocent.

But it was in the lawless town of Tombstone, Arizona, that Wyatt Earp would face his greatest challenge. As the town teetered on the brink of anarchy, torn apart by feuds and violence, Earp stepped forward to restore order, forming a posse of like-minded individuals that would come to be known as the "Earp Vendetta Ride."

In the infamous gunfight at the O.K. Corral, Wyatt Earp and his posse faced off against a band of outlaws in a showdown that would go down in history as one of the most legendary confrontations of the Wild

West. Though outnumbered and outgunned, Earp and his men emerged victorious, striking a blow against lawlessness and cementing their place in the annals of American folklore.

But Wyatt Earp's legacy extended far beyond the streets of Tombstone. As a deputy marshal and later as a gambler and entrepreneur, he continued to uphold the law and seek justice wherever he went, earning a reputation as a fearless defender of the innocent and a staunch opponent of corruption and tyranny.

And though the days of the Wild West may have long since passed, the legend of Wyatt Earp lives on—the enduring power of courage, integrity, and the unwavering pursuit of justice.

90. The Gambler's Gun

Imagine a man whose reputation was as sharp as his wit and as deadly as his aim. His name was John Henry "Doc" Holliday, a legendary figure whose skill with a deck of cards was matched only by his prowess with a pistol.

Born into a life of privilege in Georgia, Doc Holliday was trained as a dentist, earning the nickname "Doc" for his profession. But it was his love of gambling and his quick temper that would ultimately define his legacy.

Fleeing his past and seeking a new start in the rough-and-tumble frontier town of Tombstone, Arizona, Doc Holliday quickly made a name for himself as a fearsome gunslinger and a formidable opponent at the poker table. With his sharp wit and icy demeanor, he struck fear into the hearts of his adversaries, earning a reputation as one of the deadliest men in the West.

But it was his role in the infamous gunfight at the O.K. Corral that would cement Doc Holliday's place in history. In October 1881, tensions between the lawmen of Tombstone and a band of outlaws reached a boiling point, culminating in a shootout that would go down as one of the most legendary confrontations of the Wild West. Though outnumbered and outgunned, Doc Holliday and his fellow lawmen emerged victorious, striking a blow against lawlessness and cementing their place in the annals of American folklore.

But for Doc Holliday, the victory would be short-lived. Stricken with tuberculosis and haunted by his past, he would spend his remaining years on the run, a shadow of his former self.

91. The Southern Pacific Heist

In the heart of the rugged American West, where the vast expanse of nature stretched as far as the eye could see, there lay a trail of iron that carried with it the lifeblood of a nation—the Southern Pacific Railroad. And it was along this steel ribbon that one of the most audacious train robberies in history would unfold.

It was a hot September day in 1876 when the Southern Pacific train, laden with gold bullion and bound for the bustling metropolis of San Francisco, chugged its way across the arid landscape of Southern California. Little did the passengers know that they were about to become unwitting participants in a crime that would go down in infamy.

As the train rumbled along its route, a band of masked bandits lay in wait, hidden among the scrub brush and rocky outcrops that lined the tracks. Armed to the teeth and fueled by greed, they sprang into action as the train rounded a bend, its whistle piercing the stillness of the desert air.

With guns blazing and voices raised in a chorus of defiance, the outlaws stormed the train, overwhelming the crew and passengers alike with their sheer audacity. In a matter of minutes, they had secured their prize—the gold bullion that lay locked away in the train's cargo hold.

But their victory would be short-lived. As word of the robbery spread, a posse of lawmen and vigilantes was quickly assembled, hot on the trail of the fleeing bandits. And though the outlaws managed to evade capture for a time, justice would eventually catch up with them, as one by one they were hunted down and brought to justice.

Yet even as the dust settled and the stolen gold was returned to its rightful owners, the legend of the Southern Pacific heist would live on—a testament to the daring and audacity of those who dared to defy the law in pursuit of their own twisted version of the American dream.

92. The Race for a Dream

In the vast expanse of the Oklahoma Territory the promise of a new beginning beckoned like a siren's call. It was 1899 and Oklahoma Land Rush was about to begin. It was a race against time and against each other as thousands of settlers descended upon the unclaimed lands, each eager to stake their claim and build a new life on the fertile soil of the prairie.

As the sun rose on that fateful day, the air crackled with anticipation and the sound of hooves thundered across the plains. Men, women, and children from all walks of life lined up along the border, their eyes fixed on the horizon as the seconds ticked away.

And then, with a mighty roar, the starting gun sounded, and the rush was on. Wagons rattled and horses galloped as settlers raced across the open prairie, their hearts pounding with excitement and determination. With stakes in hand and dreams in their hearts, they fought through dust clouds and chaos, each determined to claim their piece of the American dream.

For some, the journey would end in triumph as they secured prime parcels of land and began to build the foundations of a new life. For others, the race would end in disappointment as they arrived too late or found themselves thwarted by obstacles along the way.

But amidst the chaos and the competition, there was a sense of camaraderie and community that bound the settlers together. Neighbors helped neighbors, strangers became friends, and together they began the arduous task of building a new society from the ground up.

The pioneering spirit of the American people and the enduring belief that with hard work, determination, and a little bit of luck, anything is possible, still lives on today.

93. The Preacher's Stand

In the dirt-choked streets of Dusty Creek, the sun beat down mercilessly on the small frontier town. Reverend John Baxter stepped off the stagecoach, his worn boots hitting the wooden boards with purpose. His mission was clear—to bring the word of God to the lawless souls of the West.

However, the townsfolk eyed him with suspicion as he made his way to the makeshift church. They were a hardened bunch, used to settling their disputes with lead rather than prayer. Yet, Baxter was undeterred, his faith unshakable.

As he preached from the pulpit, his words rang out across the empty pews. Some listened intently, while others scoffed and jeered. But Baxter persisted, his voice rising above the din.

Outside, trouble brewed. The local saloon owner, a man with a crooked smile and a quick trigger finger, saw the preacher as a threat to his way of life. He rallied his men, determined to run Baxter out of town.

That night, as Baxter lay in his bedroll, he heard the distant sound of hooves approaching. He knew trouble was coming, but he refused to back down. With a prayer on his lips, he prepared to face whatever lay ahead.

As the outlaws descended on the church, Baxter stood his ground, his Bible clutched tightly in his hand. In the ensuing chaos, shots rang out, echoing through the night. But when the dust settled, it was Baxter who emerged victorious, his faith unbroken.

In the days that followed, the people of Dusty Creek came to respect the preacher who had stood up to evil and prevailed. And though the road ahead would be long and fraught with danger, Baxter knew that he had found his calling on the frontier.

94. The Last Ride

The sun beat down mercilessly on the arid plains of Texas as the stagecoach rumbled along the dusty trail, its wheels kicking up clouds of dust in its wake. Inside, the passengers clung to their seats, their nerves on edge as they watched the horizon for signs of danger.

And then, like a bolt from the blue, the outlaws struck. Masked and armed to the teeth, they rode out of the shadows, their guns blazing as they surrounded the stagecoach and forced it to a halt. With shouts and threats, they demanded the passengers hand over their valuables, their faces twisted into cruel smiles as they plundered the carriage.

But their triumph would be short-lived. For unbeknownst to them, a posse of Texas Rangers lay in wait, hidden among the rocks and scrub brush that lined the trail. With nerves of steel and a determination to uphold the law, they sprang into action, their guns blazing as they confronted the outlaws in a hail of bullets and gunfire.

Caught off guard and outnumbered, the outlaws fought bravely but were no match for the Rangers' superior firepower and skill. One by one, they fell, their cries of defiance drowned out by the roar of gunfire and the shouts of the lawmen.

And then, in a moment of triumph and relief, the battle was over. The outlaws lay dead or wounded, their reign of terror brought to an end by the swift and decisive action of the Texas Rangers. And though the stagecoach may have been robbed, justice had prevailed.

95. The Gambler's Hand

In the dimly lit saloon of a dusty Western town, the air was thick with smoke and tension as a group of rugged men gathered around a weathered table, their eyes fixed on the glinting dice in the center. At the heart of the commotion stood Two-Fingered Morgan, the notorious gambler whose luck was as legendary as his ruthlessness.

As the stakes rose higher with each roll of the dice, the tension in the room became palpable, the sound of clinking glasses and murmured whispers fading into the background as all eyes remained fixed on the game unfolding before them. Gold and silver coins changed hands with lightning speed, fortunes won and lost in the blink of an eye as the dice danced across the table.

But it was not just the promise of riches that kept the men glued to their seats—it was the thrill of the game itself, the rush of adrenaline that came with each roll of the dice and the knowledge that at any moment, fortunes could change in an instant.

As the night wore on and the stakes climbed ever higher, the tension reached a fever pitch. Sweat beaded on brows and hearts raced in chests as the final roll of the dice approached, the outcome hanging in the balance like a knife-edge.

And then, with a flick of the wrist and a roll of the dice, the moment of truth arrived. The room held its breath as the dice clattered to a stop, revealing the winning combination in a flurry of cheers and groans.

For some, it was a night of triumph and celebration, their pockets bulging with ill-gotten gains. But for others, it was a bitter defeat, their hopes dashed in an instant by the cruel hand of fate.

Yet as the night drew to a close and the players drifted away into the darkness, there remained a sense of camaraderie and respect among them—a shared bond forged in the heat of battle and the thrill of the game. And though they may have parted ways as rivals, they would forever be united by the memory of that high-stakes dice game in the heart of the Wild West.

96. A Wagon Driver's Peril

In the rugged hills of the Colorado Rockies, where the wind whispered secrets of silver and gold, Old Joe made his living as a two-horse wagon driver, ferrying precious cargo to and from the mines that dotted the landscape. But it was on one fateful day, as he made his way down the treacherous mountain roads with the mine payroll in tow, that his skills would be put to the ultimate test.

With his trusty team of horses, Thunder and Lightning, Old Joe navigated the winding trails with practiced ease, his eyes scanning the horizon for any sign of trouble. But as he rounded a bend in the road, he was greeted by a sight that made his blood run cold—a band of masked bandits, their guns trained on him and their intentions clear.

Thinking quickly, Old Joe spurred his horses into action, urging them to greater speed as he raced down the mountain, the sound of gunfire echoing in his ears. Bullets whizzed past him, kicking up clouds of dust as Thunder and Lightning galloped towards safety, their hooves pounding against the rocky terrain.

But just as it seemed they might escape, disaster struck. With a deafening crack, a stray bullet found its mark, striking Lightning in the flank and sending him tumbling to the ground in a cloud of dust and pain.

With a heavy heart, Old Joe leapt from the wagon and drew his gun, ready to defend the payroll with his life if need be. But to his surprise, the bandits had vanished as quickly as they had appeared, leaving him alone on the mountain with his wounded horse and the precious cargo he had sworn to protect.

Gritting his teeth against the pain of loss and determination burning in his heart, Old Joe lifted Lightning onto the wagon and continued on his journey, his eyes fixed on the horizon as he vowed to deliver the payroll, come hell or high water.

97. The Saloon Showdown

In the heart of a dusty frontier town, the Silver Dollar Saloon stood as a symbol of both camaraderie and conflict. It was a place where cowboys and miners gathered to drink away their troubles, but also where simmering tensions between rival factions often boiled over into violence.

On this particular evening, the air in the saloon was thick with tension as the Hatfield gang and the McCoy boys squared off across the room, their eyes smoldering with hatred and resentment. It was no secret that these two factions had been at odds for years, feuding over territory, cattle, and the affections of a local beauty named Rose.

As the night wore on and tempers flared, a single spark was all it took to ignite the powder keg of hostility that had been building for so long. Insults were hurled, fists flew, and before anyone knew it, the saloon erupted into chaos.

Tables were overturned, bottles smashed, and chairs splintered as the rival factions clashed with a ferocity that threatened to tear the building apart. The sound of breaking glass and gunfire filled the air, mingling with the shouts and screams of the terrified patrons caught in the crossfire.

But amidst the chaos, a lone figure emerged—a stranger with a badge pinned to his chest and a six-shooter at his hip. With nerves of steel and a voice like thunder, he called for order, demanding that the feuding factions lay down their arms and settle their differences like men.

And miraculously, they listened. With a mixture of relief and shame, the Hatfields and McCoys lowered their weapons, their eyes meeting across the smoky haze of the saloon. And as they shook hands and shared a drink in the aftermath of the confrontation, they knew that, for now at least, peace had been restored to the Silver Dollar Saloon.

98. The Shadows of El Dorado

Amidst the dust-choked streets of El Dorado, a golden fever coursed through the veins of every soul. Miners from far and wide converged upon the town, drawn by the promise of untold riches buried beneath its sun-baked soil.

In the midst of this frenzy stood John Morgan, a seasoned prospector with a heart as weathered as the parched landscape. For years, he had toiled in the shadows of the Sierra Nevada, scraping a meager existence from the earth. But now, with the discovery of gold, his dreams of wealth seemed within reach.

Yet, as the veins of ore ran deeper, so too did the currents of greed and betrayal. In the saloons and gambling halls, whispers of treachery and deceit echoed like the howl of a desert wind. Claims were disputed, friendships forged in hardship shattered by the lure of fortune.

John watched with a heavy heart as the town he once knew descended into chaos. Men once bound by camaraderie now turned against each other in a ruthless pursuit of wealth. Fistfights erupted in the streets, and the air crackled with tension like a tinderbox waiting to ignite.

But amidst the chaos, John remained steadfast in his resolve. He knew that true riches lay not in the glittering veins of gold, but in the bonds of trust and loyalty forged in the crucible of adversity. And so, with grit and determination, he vowed to protect what remained of his town, even as the shadows of greed threatened to consume it whole.

99. Unmasking the Medicine Show

In the heart of the frontier town of Newton, anticipation rippled through the dusty streets as the arrival of the traveling medicine show loomed on the horizon. For the townsfolk, weary from the hardships of pioneer life, the promise of miracle cures and captivating entertainment was a beacon of hope in an otherwise harsh existence.

Led by the enigmatic Dr. Ezekiel Stone, the medicine show descended upon Newton like a whirlwind of color and excitement, its wagons adorned with flamboyant banners and flashing lights. With a silver tongue and a charming smile, Dr. Stone captivated the crowd with tales of miraculous healings and wondrous remedies, promising relief from ailments both real and imagined.

But as the days passed and the initial excitement waned, whispers began to circulate among the townsfolk, casting doubt on the authenticity of Dr. Stone's claims. Rumors of mysterious disappearances and unexplained illnesses followed in the wake of the medicine show, sowing seeds of suspicion and fear among the residents of Newton.

Determined to uncover the truth, a group of concerned citizens banded together, led by the town sheriff and local doctor. Their investigation unearthed a dark secret hidden beneath the veneer of Dr. Stone's charismatic facade—a trail of deception and deceit stretching back for years.

In a dramatic confrontation, the truth was revealed, and Dr. Stone's true identity as a charlatan and fraudster was laid bare for all to see. With the support of the townsfolk, the authorities apprehended the impostors, bringing an end to their nefarious scheme and restoring peace to the once-troubled streets of Newton.

As the medicine show wagons rolled out of town, the residents of Newton breathed a collective sigh of relief, grateful to have escaped the clutches of deception and fraud. And though the scars of betrayal would linger, they emerged stronger and more united than ever, ready to face whatever challenges the frontier had in store.

100. The Phantom's Gambit

In the serene township of North Fork, where the sun dipped low on the horizon, casting long shadows over the quiet streets, a gang of notorious outlaws descended upon the local bank. Led by the infamous outlaw known as "The Phantom," they struck with ruthless precision, their faces hidden behind masks as they emptied the vault of its riches.

The news of the brazen bank robbery spread like wildfire through North Fork, sending shockwaves of fear and uncertainty rippling through the community. But amidst the chaos, one man stood resolute against the tide of lawlessness – the town's stalwart sheriff, Lucas McCain.

With a determined glint in his eye and a Winchester rifle at his side, Sheriff McCain vowed to bring "The Phantom" and his gang to justice, no matter the cost. As the outlaws made their daring escape, he embarked on a relentless pursuit, tracking them through the rugged wilderness of the frontier.

What followed was a deadly game of cat and mouse, as Sheriff McCain and his posse clashed with the outlaws in a series of thrilling showdowns across the unforgiving terrain of the Wild West. With each passing day, tensions mounted and the stakes grew higher, as the fate of North Fork hung in the balance.

But in the end, it was Sheriff McCain who emerged victorious, his unwavering determination and unwavering courage leading to the capture of "The Phantom" and his gang. As the outlaws were brought to justice, the townsfolk of North Fork breathed a collective sigh of relief, knowing that their beloved town was safe once more.

And though the scars of the bank robbery would linger, they served as a testament to the bravery and resilience of the people of North Fork, who refused to cower in the face of adversity and stood tall in the fight for justice.

101. Trail of Endurance

In the rugged town of Frontier Falls, Sheriff Paul Forrester squared off against the notorious outlaw, "Desperado" Dan Smith, in a tense showdown that would decide the fate of the lawless town. With the sun high in the sky and tensions escalating by the second, the dusty streets became the stage for a thrilling confrontation.

As the clock struck high noon, Sheriff Forrester and "Desperado" Dan faced each other, their eyes locked in a silent battle of wills. The townsfolk held their breath, knowing that this showdown would determine whether law and order would prevail or chaos would reign unchecked.

With a lightning-fast draw, the gunslingers unleashed a barrage of bullets, the echoes of gunfire reverberating through the streets. Dust billowed around them as they dodged and weaved, each shot a deadly reminder of the stakes of their confrontation.

As the duel reached its climax, Sheriff Forrester's steady aim proved true, and "Desperado" Dan fell to the ground, defeated but not forgotten. The townsfolk erupted into cheers as Sheriff Forrester holstered his weapon, his victory a testament to the courage and determination of those who stood on the side of justice.

In the aftermath of the showdown, Frontier Falls breathed a sigh of relief, knowing that Sheriff Forrester's bravery had saved their town from the clutches of lawlessness. And though the scars of their encounter would linger, they served as a reminder of the price of freedom and the sacrifices made to protect it.

The End

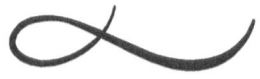

101 Western Short Stories -
Jamie Stonebridge, Sam Suncroft
Copyright © 2024
Seniority / Everbreeze Media Oy
This is a work of fiction. Names and characters are the product of the author's imagination and any resemblance to actual persons, living or dead, is entirely coincidental.
Set in 16.5 pt EB Garamond

www.ingramcontent.com/pod-product-compliance
Lightning Source LLC
Chambersburg PA
CBHW020647220526
45464CB00001B/327